HIV/AIDS in Latin American Countries

The Challenges Ahead

Human Development Network
Health, Nutrition, and Population Series

HIV/AIDS in Latin American Countries

The Challenges Ahead

Anabela Garcia Abreu
Isabel Noguer
Karen Cowgill

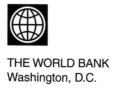

THE WORLD BANK
Washington, D.C.

Library of Congress Cataloging-in-Publication Data

HIV/AIDS in Latin America : the challenges ahead / Anabela Garcia-Abreu, Isabel
    Noguer, Karen Cowgill [editors].
      p. cm.—(Health, nutrition, and population series)
    Includes bibliographical references.
    ISBN 0-8213-5364-0
      1. AIDS (Disease)—Latin America. I. Garcia-Abreu, Anabela, 1955-II. Noguer, Isabel, 1956-
III. Cowgill, Karen, 1967-IV. Series.

RA643.86.L29H585 2003
362.1'969792'0098—dc21   2003052529

Contents

Tables

Figures

Preface

Compared with most countries in Africa, and with the nearby islands of the Caribbean, many Latin American countries have not faced a full-scale AIDS epidemic. On average, Latin American countries estimate HIV prevalence among 15- to 49-year-olds at 0.5 percent. Around 130,000 adults and children were newly infected with HIV during 2001, and 80,000 died. Although AIDS accounts for only a fraction of all adult deaths in most Latin American nations, those deaths occur in the most productive years of life. There are worrisome signs in several countries in the Region; the disease appears to be evolving—from affecting virtually only the highest risk groups, such as men who have sex with men (MSM) and injecting drug users (IDUs)—to becoming an increasingly generalized problem. Throughout the Region, many behaviors associated with the spread of HIV/AIDS (young age at first intercourse, violence against women, injecting drug use) are commonplace, and with the exception of a small number of countries, the response to the threat of HIV/AIDS has been slow, small-scale, and largely only supported by external agencies and international programs. If the warning signs are heeded, and appropriate prevention measures are taken in the very near future, Latin America has the opportunity to avoid the sad stories seen in other parts of the world.

Sound and timely policies can limit the current and future impact of HIV/AIDS on Latin American health care systems, economies, and societies. Good policies are based on understanding the scope and special nature of the HIV/AIDS problem, and confronting it in a way that respects human rights.

This book attempts to present new and updated information about the extent and trends of the HIV/AIDS epidemic in Latin America; to evaluate current national surveillance capacity; to assess national responses of the health sector to the epidemic on a country-by-country basis; to identify key areas in which specific interventions are urgently needed; and to outline the challenges ahead.

Rich in information, and based on both analyses of secondary information and a full set of newly collected country-level data, this book is intended to be the basis for discussions within and across countries, and between countries of the Region and their development partners.

This study was conducted in 2001 and included 17 countries: Argentina, Bolivia, Brazil, Chile, Colombia, Costa Rica, Ecuador, El Salvador, Guatemala, Honduras, Mexico, Nicaragua, Panama, Paraguay, Peru, República Bolivariana de Venezuela, and Uruguay.

It would be worthwhile for the World Bank, as well as the countries themselves, to conduct a form of self-evaluation in terms of the achievements, obstacles, and challenges ahead; and it would be very useful to make this information available to all actors involved. In the future, this study could become a point of departure for comparing this year's results to others. If the report were to be made publicly available, countries and institutions could use it for their own evaluation.

For purposes of analysis, some countries were aggregated into subregions, according to similarities in socioeconomic level, health system, and epidemiological pattern of the epidemic; geographical proximity; economic, cultural, and politic interests; cultural roots; and frequency of internal migrations. Three subregions were analyzed: Central America (Costa Rica, El Salvador, Guatemala, Honduras, Nicaragua, and Panama); the Andean Region (Bolivia, Colombia, Ecuador, Peru, and República Bolivariana de Venezuela); and the Southern Cone (Argentina, Chile, Paraguay, and Uruguay).

Brazil and Mexico were analyzed individually. Both countries possess much higher resources; their national programs have reached a high level of development; and the disease's epidemiological pattern presents some characteristics seen in industrialized countries.

The study uses primary and secondary data. *Primary data* were collected using four survey instruments specifically geared to this study. The surveys were designed to assess surveillance systems and national responses to the epidemic from the health sector. Before distribution to the target group of respondents, the survey instruments were reviewed by experts working in the field who had knowledge of the Latin America region.*

Data on surveillance systems were collected through a self-administered, semi-structured questionnaire applied to those managing national HIV/AIDS surveillance systems in 17 Latin American countries (i.e., technicians from the national AIDS program or from the departments of epidemiology, depending on the countries). The survey instrument included questions assessing the case definition, reporting procedures, type of surveillance, sources of information, and feedback of the surveillance information. All countries surveyed sent in their questionnaires, but the level of completion of the questionnaires was variable.

Data on the institutional capacity to fight the epidemic were collected using three questionnaires. These questionnaires were given to the heads of national HIV/AIDS programs, to key respondents from nongovernmental organizations (NGOs), and to physicians working in the field. Most physician and NGO questionnaires were completed face-to-face by trained interviewers.

In each country a questionnaire was given to the director of the national HIV/AIDS program. The following topics were covered in the questionnaire: (1) description of the program; (2) multisectoral coordination and legislation; (3) sensitization/prevention interventions directed to the general population and adolescents; (4) interventions targeting high-risk groups; (5) interventions for preventing

---

*These experts included HIV/AIDS specialists, a former national HIV/AIDS coordinator, a population and health specialist, a demographer, a public health specialist and an epidemiologist. The questionnaires were administered to the target group of respondents, preceded by a letter presenting the study and explaining the methodology.

mother-to-child transmission; (6) access to the health system and prevention methods; (7) financing and relations with NGOs; (8) characteristics/coverage of health and social services provided; (9) relations with international agencies; and (10) main problems faced in controlling the epidemic in that country.

NGOs were selected according to the following criteria: years of experience and level of integration in the countries (favoring those with larger history in the fight against HIV/AIDS); whether they were community-based, working with high-risk groups or people living with HIV/AIDS (PLWHA); and implementation of various HIV/AIDS-related activities (prevention, psychological, legal, and social support). Eighty-four NGOs were selected from a pool of more than 900. Among the NGOs surveyed, the average period of working with HIV/AIDS patients is eight years; 60 percent of these NGOs work at the national level, serving over 500,000 people in the Region. In all, 4,000 people work for the NGOs surveyed (this includes full-time and part-time workers and volunteers).

The NGO questionnaire was designed to cover the following aspects: characteristics of the NGO (level of integration, resources, work environment, target populations, involvement in networks, and objectives of the organization); activities over the last year regarding HIV/AIDS, specifying target populations, budget, flow of funds, and coverage and impact of the interventions; level of coordination with governments and national plans; status of the epidemic and those affected from the perspective of the NGO; and main problems and obstacles (present and future) for controlling the epidemic.

Physicians were selected according to the following criteria: significant experience in clinical management of patients with HIV/AIDS, and experience working in large health facilities.

Five physicians were selected from each country; these were recommended by national HIV/AIDS programs and by experts from the Region. Sixty-four (75.3 percent) agreed to contribute information and opinions for this study. The 64 physicians surveyed have, on average, 13 years of experience in the clinical management of patients with HIV/AIDS—more than half (59 percent) in both public and private practice—and serve approximately 50 patients per month.

The physician questionnaire focused on history (years in the current health sector and level of professional experience); conditions under which she/he practices (good-practice protocols, conditions for diagnosing and treating patients); coverage of basic services for diagnosing and treating patients; knowledge of HIV/AIDS in the population; and issues with infrastructure and health care resources for effectively controlling the epidemic.

Secondary data were drawn from national statistics and were complemented by data published by international organizations (WHO/PAHO, UNAIDS, and SIDALAC), and data from studies conducted in the Region and identified through databases, as well as from national strategic plans.

National surveillance systems provided data on incidence and prevalence of HIV and AIDS. From the same sources, the study used data on incidence and prevalence of STIs and HIV in different sentinel populations (blood donors, CSWs, MSM, IDUs, and others).

Certain countries are not included in certain tables and charts, which indicates that the corresponding relevant data were not available.

This document touches upon the broader context in which the response to HIV/AIDS in Latin America is taking place; however, it focuses more specifically on how the health-sector response is seen by different country players. Results and conclusions drawn from this study represent the views and opinions of a group of key respondents selected from the national HIV/AIDS programs, NGOs, and physicians; these were supplemented with information from other sources. Therefore, these views cannot be and were not extrapolated or generalized to the overall national response of a country.

Acknowledgments

This study was prepared by Anabela Garcia Abreu (Task Team Leader), Isabel Noguer, and Karen Cowgill (consultants). Girindre Beharry and Ruth Levine (LCSHD), Paloma Cuchí (UNAIDS /PAHO), José Izazola-Licea (SIDALAC), and Nicolas Noriega-Portilla (economist) also provided written contributions. Pilar Ramón tabulated the data collected through questionnaires. Special thanks to Marian Kaminskis for her substantial input, editorial, and logistics assistance, as well as to Natalia Moncada for her follow-up on the final phase. Our thanks also to Madalena Cabeçadas for her technical input.

Julia del Amo, Maria José Belza, James Cercone, Fiorella Salazar, Laura Altobelli (consultants), Claudia Macías, Magdalena Colmenares, Sandra Cesilini (World Bank), and María Etelvina Barros (UNAIDS) administered the questionnaires.

Peer reviewers of the study include: Charles Griffin and Martha Aisworth (World Bank), Fernando Zacarías (PAHO), Luis Loures and Enrique Zelaya (UNAIDS), and Richard Keenlyside (CDC). Peer reviewers of the questionnaires were: Sandra Rosenhouse, Gerard la Forgia, Michele Gragnolati (World Bank), and José Izazola-Licea (SIDALAC).

Special thanks to all who took the time to complete the questionnaires. They are truly the key people who made this study possible: the national program directors, NGOs, and physicians (listed in Appendix 2).

The team would like to extend its gratitude to UNAIDS and PAHO, in both headquarters and local offices, for their help in identifying the key informants and arranging the logistics of the distribution of the questionnaires, helping with data collection, and for providing pertinent bibliographic sources. Our thanks also to Spanish International Cooperation for helping with data collection, especially in Latin American countries.

Executive Summary

Although the risk behaviors and biological markers that fuel the epidemic are widespread, many Latin American countries have not yet faced a full-scale AIDS epidemic. On average, Latin American countries estimate HIV prevalence among 15- to 49-year-olds at 0.5 percent. Around 130,000 adults and children were infected with HIV in 2001, and 80,000 died of AIDS.

HIV/AIDS in Latin America falls within the framework of a low endemic setting. In the majority of the countries, the epidemic is still concentrated in high-risk populations: men who have sex with men (MSM), injecting drug users (IDUs), commercial sex workers (CSWs), prisoners, and people with sexually transmitted infections (STIs). The exceptions are Honduras and southeastern Brazil, where the epidemic has reached the general population. Heterosexual sex is the primary mode of transmission in Central America, with sex between men predominating in South America, and injecting drug use playing a significant role in the Southern Cone. Survey respondents also identified other populations with increased vulnerability in which interventions would be crucial—young people and women. Although the number of men living with AIDS outweighs the number of women in all countries, the gender gap is closing, and in some countries, the effect of AIDS on rural communities is increasing rapidly.

In low endemic settings, the main priority is the highest risk groups, and activities to address HIV/AIDS should be focused on

(1) strengthening efforts to prevent new infections in these populations, and (2) providing care and support strategies, which in turn create incentives for early detection of infection and/or risky behavior.

Epidemiological surveillance plays a key role in the control of the epidemic through the measurement of frequency, distribution, and evolution of HIV/AIDS among populations; identification of high-risk groups; and evaluation of the effectiveness of prevention efforts.

In Latin America, epidemiological surveillance of HIV/AIDS at the national level began in the 1980s. Since then, allocation of resources and personnel has steadily increased, leading to well-established surveillance systems based on AIDS cases notification. Presently, in every Latin American country, the reporting of AIDS cases is mandatory. However there are persistent high levels of underreporting and delays in reporting. The epidemic in Latin America is likely to include around 30 percent more cases of AIDS and 40 percent more cases of HIV than currently estimated.

Since the late 1980s, Latin American countries have demonstrated the capacity to confront the HIV/AIDS epidemic, developing new structures and the groundwork needed for community responses.

At the global level, there have been continuous efforts to mobilize political leadership at the highest levels of national, regional, and global governance. At the country level, much has been achieved. By the end of 2001, almost all countries in Latin America had their national strategic frameworks finalized or were in the process of completion. In most cases, the plans were developed with participation from a broad range of stakeholders (including various government ministries, civil society, associations of people living with HIV/AIDS, bilateral and multilateral partners), and they now serve as the common reference for action. The national strategic plan process also resulted in a clear shift in the perception of the epidemic from a health-only issue to a broader social and developmental approach.

Latin America has an excellent basis for effective interventions with multilateral and/or bilateral organizations. The resources infrastructure and professionals are in place to implement a variety of interventions, evaluate their impact, and sustain them over time.

However, the capacity to respond has been limited by political, technical, and social problems. The challenge ahead is to tackle some of the chronic problems that affect the national response.

Results from this study bring to light many aspects of the health sector response to the HIV epidemic that could be improved and they provide feasible prioritized solutions. The study unravels the gains from an expanded response by engaging much more closely the community and social movements around HIV/AIDS.

In terms of the health sector, this study identified several key problems and offered possible solutions.

Prevention

Key Problems

In the national response there are insufficient interventions targeting high-risk groups, worsened by a substantial lack of information on the magnitude and trend of the epidemic. These include MSM, CSWs, IDUs, and other groups such as prisoners. Health and sexual education programs for adolescents and young people are widespread but the skills to prevent HIV infection in these groups may be lacking from its content. Levels of multisectoral coordination are unequal among countries in the Region. Although there are structures in place to foster multisectoral coordination in almost all countries, the level of true collaboration is still low, lacking resources and adequate coverage for coordinated execution of interventions. At the same time, there is limited coordination between NGOs and governments in interventions for specific populations. NGOs are much more likely to have access to marginal populations, or those that lack health services, yet governments and most NGOs dedicate the majority of their efforts to groups with "variable risk" for infection (i.e. the general population, young people, women, etc.). A stronger and continuous involvement from civil society needs to be ensured, since it may be the only way to expand the response to AIDS in the near future.

How to Address them?

- Enhance approaches that focus on social mobilization and on building up of community responses.

- Improve multisectoral coordination.

- Intensify interventions for high-risk groups, where HIV infection reaches the highest levels.

- Promote gender policies that strengthen and build equitable relationships.

Access to Health and Social Services

Key Problems

In Latin America, a substantial number of people infected with HIV do not have access to adequate and comprehensive health care. The reasons for this are diverse, including limited access to services and below-quality standards. Insufficient medical training is one of the main deficiencies impacting health care, along with lack of appropriate clinical management guidelines. Finally, access to new antiretroviral therapies is hindered due to cost and health infrastructure.

There are general deficiencies, such as the need to strengthen resources infrastructure, especially the network of HIV diagnostic laboratories, labs for determining CD4 levels* and viral load†, as well as infrastructure needed for diagnosis and follow-up for coinciding infections and other disease processes associated with HIV. According to national programs, the network of laboratories is insufficient, especially in Central America and the Andean Region (although this

---

*CD4 count refers to a measure of "helper" T cells that help B cells produce antibodies. The number of CD4 cells is an important measure of an individual's immune system capabilities.

†Viral load test is a measure of the amount of HIV in the blood to determine how far infection has progressed.

is characteristic of all Latin America). Access to services is limited by the payment required.

Substantial numbers of people are unaware that they are infected by HIV. Barriers that prevent greater coverage and have implications for supply and demand (such as discrimination, confidentiality, etc.) prevent people from coming early to the services. There is also the need to pay more attention to those interventions for decreasing mother-to-child transmission of HIV in health centers.

How to Address them?

- Improve health and social services through multisectoral collaboration.

- Promote HIV testing, especially among high-risk populations.

- Offer HIV testing to all pregnant women.

- Strengthen health infrastructure and laboratory networks.

- Train physicians and nurses in clinical management and treatment of HIV and other STIs.

Human Rights

Key Problems

Lack of information, stigmatization, homophobia, and social prejudices regarding sexual orientation or behavior prevent access to prevention and clinical care in Latin America. These are some of the obstacles that people at high-risk or who are infected face when trying to access services. These also hinder access of people living with HIV and AIDS (PLWHA), which impedes fair and equitable treatment.

How to Address them?

- Fight against ignorance and promote human rights.

- Preserve the right to access health, social, and psychological care.

- Promote programs addressing the issue of schooling for HIV-positive children.

- Promote the right to work and integration or re-integration in the workforce.

- Involve PLWHA in all strategies for prevention and control of the epidemic.

National Capacity: Structure and Management

Key Problems

The multiplicity of health problems affecting Latin America and the health sector reforms are part of the circumstances that have prevented Latin America from giving a more articulated response to the epidemic. Most of the countries have multisectoral plans with the participation of multi-partners; however, the actual functionality and capacity for a collaborative response has been mediated by the technical and political capacity of national programs and by limited resources available for HIV/AIDS control. Stronger involvement from civil society, communities, and associations of PLWHA is critical to the response to AIDS in the Region.

Surveillance systems in Latin America need to be strengthened to provide accurate data for decision making. Availability of systematized information on the incidence of newly diagnosed HIV infections and sentinel surveillance coverage (especially among the most affected groups) is scarce throughout the Region. Registries of AIDS cases, which have the greatest tradition and permanence, show high levels of under-reporting in certain subregions, especially Central America. Currently, these systems don't provide a clear picture of the magnitude and trends of the epidemic, and they are also weak in capturing the early signs of alarm given by the dissemination of the epidemic. These systems should include a behavioral component.

How to Address them?

- Consolidate multisectoral responses to the epidemic, and bring national strategic plans into a reality.

- Strengthen epidemiological surveillance systems.

- Establish guidelines for prevention interventions and consolidate the interventions that have been most cost-effective.

- Blood safety policies should be revised to achieve universal testing of donated blood and acceptance of only voluntary, altruistic, non-remunerated donations.

- Provide continuous capacity-building of human resources.

- Increase available resources.

- Overcome cultural, social, and religious factors that obstruct good technical proposals or government decisions.

- Encourage and support NGO networks.

- Increase synergy and coordination among different actors in the Region.

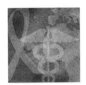

Abbreviations
and Acronyms

AIDS	Acquired immune deficiency syndrome
ARV	Antiretrovirals
CDC	Centers for Disease Control and Prevention
CSW	Commercial sex worker
HAART	Highly active antiretroviral therapy
HIV	Human immunodeficiency virus
IBRD	International Bank for Reconstruction and Development
IDUs	Injecting drug users
IFA	Immuno-florescence assay
INH	Isoniazide
MoH	Ministry of Health
MSM	Men who have sex with men
NGOs	Nongovernmental organizations
PAHO	Pan American Health Organization
PLWHA	People living with HIV/AIDS
STIs	Sexually transmitted infections
UNAIDS	Joint United Nations HIV/AIDS Program
WB	Western blot
WHO	World Health Organization

CHAPTER 1

Epidemiological Overview and Economic Impact

Summary

Accurate numbers of people living with HIV/AIDS (PLWHA) in Latin America are lacking. Underdiagnosis and underreporting contribute to inexact HIV/AIDS statistics. The best estimates by the Joint United Nations Programme on HIV/AIDS (UNAIDS), the Pan American Health Organization (PAHO), and the World Health Organization (WHO) of the number of people living with HIV/AIDS in Latin America at the end of 2001 was 1.4 million, or approximately 0.50 percent of the entire Latin American population. In Latin America, 130,000 adults and children were newly infected with HIV during 2001, and 80,000 died. WHO reported that HIV in 1999 ranked second as a cause of disability-adjusted life years in the world.

For the most part, the HIV/AIDS epidemic in Latin America is concentrated in specific high-risk groups. Although the epidemic in Latin America is still largely concentrated in males, the so-called feminization of the epidemic is evident in decreasing male-to-female ratios among those with AIDS. Injecting drug use is an important route of HIV transmission in parts of South America, especially countries in the Southern Cone, Brazil, and Colombia. Commercial sex workers (CSWs) are also at high risk of acquiring and transmitting HIV, and men who have sex with men (MSM) account for a substantial amount of HIV transmission. Patients with sexually transmitted infections (STIs) represent another high-risk group; however, the incidence is not well documented in many countries.

In Mexico, the epidemic is still largely concentrated in MSM. AIDS is the third most common cause of death in males and the sixth in females 25–44 years of age. On the other hand, HIV transmission in Central America is overwhelmingly via heterosexual sex, making it more similar to the Caribbean than to South America or Mexico. The situation in this region is serious and expected to worsen, as we see new infections in the youngest population and especially among females.

The HIV/AIDS epidemic is most heterogeneous in Brazil, where HIV has been detected in all population groups. The number of PLWHA is increasing due to the wide coverage of antiretroviral therapy. The number of PLWHA in Brazil was estimated at 540,000 at the end of 1999.

The Andean region presents evidence of a high prevalence of risky sexual behaviors; this region had the highest estimated incidence of STIs (15 percent) in all of Latin America in 1997. Over 40 percent of reported AIDS cases were attributed to sex between men, with a nearly equal number attributed to heterosexual sex. Underreporting of HIV/AIDS is probably substantial in this region because of scarce resources and weak surveillance systems.

In the Southern Cone, Argentina has the highest prevalence of HIV infection in South America and one of the highest percentages of infected children, and HIV infections are on the rise. Among reported AIDS cases, injecting drug use plays the largest role, closely followed by sex between men. While there is probably a great deal of underreporting, as in the other regions, the Southern Cone has the lowest percentage of cases with an unknown or unclassified mode of transmission of all the regions.

There are significant additional health care and societal problems caused by HIV/AIDS. For example, tuberculosis (TB) is a major problem in Latin America, and the HIV epidemic has exacerbated it.

Thirty to 50 percent of adults in Latin America are believed to have latent TB, which often takes the opportunity of decreased immunity to manifest itself. The HIV/AIDS epidemic has also had a heavy macroeconomic impact because of the high costs of treatment and lives lost, which divert resources from productive investments.

Quantifying the Epidemic

There are wide variations in the availability and reliability of HIV testing, identification of people who have progressed to AIDS, completeness and timeliness of cases reported, and epidemiological surveillance throughout Latin America (see chapter 2). Many identified HIV infections and AIDS cases are not reported to ministries of health because of inefficiency or lack of resources. Apart from the underreporting problem, the majority of PLWHA have not been tested and do not know they are infected. Some avoid being tested for fear of stigma, while others encounter barriers to testing such as high cost, lack of local availability, or bureaucratic impediments (Díez and others 2000). Some simply do not realize or will not acknowledge that they are at risk. Data regarding the magnitude of underdiagnosis are lacking, but it exists to varying degrees in all countries.

Underdiagnosis and underreporting make it difficult to interpret HIV/AIDS statistics. Statistics reported by ministries of health and PAHO, UNAIDS, and WHO are based on *reported* cases, which substantially underestimate the true number of cases. The interpretation of statistics and comparisons among countries can be misleading because reporting completeness varies and because reporting practices and protocols differ over time and within countries. In some countries both people who are infected with HIV but have no symptoms of illness *and* people whose condition has progressed to AIDS are reported to the ministry of health, while in other countries only people who have progressed to AIDS are reported. In addition, the definition of AIDS may vary within and among countries. Some countries have well-developed epidemiological surveillance systems and are able to capture the dynamics of the epidemic by actively testing sentinel populations such as pregnant women at prenatal visits or high-risk groups like CSWs, while others with fewer resources rely on reports that trickle in from field offices.

Data are generated by research studies undertaken by government, nongovernment, or academic institutions in many countries in Latin America. While these studies may be valid for the populations in which they are conducted, applying the results to the general population may be problematic. If such studies are carried out in urban areas and among groups at high risk for HIV infection, they are likely to overestimate the true number of cases.

Given the difficulties in quantifying the HIV/AIDS epidemic from these data, PAHO, UNAIDS, and WHO have been working together on estimates of the number of people living with HIV/AIDS in Latin America (*HIV and AIDS in the Americas* 2001). These estimates of the prevalence of HIV and AIDS by country are the midpoints of ranges obtained from projections that incorporate assumptions about the incidence and progression of HIV infection. While these estimates are not necessarily accurate in an absolute sense (they are likely to overestimate the true prevalence), combined with the classification of the epidemic's status they provide the best relative measure of the HIV/AIDS epidemic in each country. The uncertainties inherent in the figures reported here do not make them invalid. The HIV/AIDS epidemic is constantly evolving and cannot be quantified in precise, static terms.

UNAIDS, WHO, and PAHO have developed guidelines for characterizing the status of the epidemic (UNAIDS 2000n) and have published estimates of HIV prevalence by country (UNAIDS 2000k).[1] The guidelines classify epidemics as low level, concentrated, or generalized based on HIV prevalence in pregnant women and in high-risk subpopulations such as injecting drug users (IDUs), MSM, and CSWs.

The purpose of this chapter is to describe, within the limits of the available data for this study, the current status of the HIV/AIDS epidemic, particular groups affected, and the adoption of prevention and treatment efforts in each of 17 Latin American countries, the Latin American region as a whole, and the subregions of Central America, the Andean Region, and the Southern Cone. This chapter and the country fact sheets in Appendix 1 draw heavily on estimates generated by PAHO, UNAIDS, and WHO, as well as on other UNAIDS documents, the strategic plans and assessments of the region's ministries of health, published reports in the medical literature, conference abstracts, and the results of our survey of key professionals in each country. The figures given in this report should be taken as relative indicators of the magnitude and severity of a dynamic epidemic.

HIV/AIDS in Latin America

The best estimate of the number of PLWHA in Latin America at the end of 2001 was 1.4 million, or approximately 0.50 percent of the Latin American population (PAHO 2001a). In 2001, 130,000 adults and children were newly infected with HIV, and 80,000 died. WHO reported that HIV was the second leading cause of disability-adjusted life years (DALYs) in the world in 1999 (Michaud, Murray, and Bloom 2001). A 1990 estimate of the burden of HIV/AIDS in Latin America and the Caribbean put total DALYs in males at 233,000 and in females at 850,000 (Murray and López 1998). Table 1.1 lists HIV/AIDS-related statistics for 1999 by country.

For the most part, the HIV/AIDS epidemic in Latin America is concentrated in specific high-risk groups. Exceptions are Honduras and southeastern Brazil, where the epidemic has reached the general population.[1] Heterosexual sex is the main mode of transmission in Central America; in South America sex between men dominates; and injecting drug use plays a significant role in the Southern Cone. The number of males living with AIDS exceeds the number of females in all countries, but the gender gap is closing.

The so-called feminization of the epidemic is evident in decreasing male-to-female ratios among those with AIDS and increasing rates of HIV infection in pregnant women and children. Increasing cases of AIDS and HIV infection identified among women in their 20s suggest that adolescent girls are at high risk. The majority of both boys and girls report their first sexual encounters in their teens or, in

Table 1.1. HIV Prevalence, AIDS Incidence, and Mortality from AIDS by Country, 1999

COUNTRY	ESTIMATED HIV PREVALENCE IN 15- TO 49-YEAR-OLDS (%)	REPORTED AIDS CASES	REPORTED AIDS INCIDENCE PER MILLION INHABITANTS	ESTIMATED DEATHS FROM AIDS	ESTIMATED AIDS MORTALITY PER MILLION INHABITANTS
Mexico	0.3	4,372	42	4,204	48
Guatemala	1.4	730	66	3,600	325
El Salvador	0.6	425	69	1,300	211
Honduras	1.9	1,136	180	4,200	665
Nicaragua	0.2	36	8	360	73
Costa Rica	0.5	215	58	750	191
Panama	1.5	534	190	1,200	427
Brazil	0.6	18,288	109	18,000	107
Venezuela, R. B. de	0.5	—	—	2,000	84
Colombia	0.3	547[a]	13	1,473	35
Ecuador	0.3	325	26	1,400	113
Peru	0.4	1,009	40	4,100	163
Bolivia	0.1	21	3[b]	380	47
Argentina	0.7	1,401	38	1,800	49
Paraguay	0.1	49	9	220	41
Uruguay	0.4	172	53	150	45
Chile	0.2	518	34	1,000	67
Total	0.5	29,325	62	46,860	99

— Not available.
Note: Prevalence is the percentage of people infected out of the entire population at risk, and incidence is the rate of new cases in a specified population over a defined period.
a. This figure is approximately half that reported in previous years.
b. This figure is 6, according to the country report.
Source: UNAIDS 2000k, PAHO 2001a, and original survey data.

some cases, their preteens. Boys are at lower risk of infection from this early sexual activity because they tend to have partners nearer their own age who are less likely to be infected with HIV. Encouraging reports indicate that youths in some countries in the region are increasingly likely to have used a condom during their first sex act (*HIV and AIDS in the Americas* 2001). However, almost half of the females and a quarter of the males in a sample of over 600 adolescents and young adults in Lima, Peru, reported being coerced into having sexual relations. Those who were coerced at their first encounter were more likely to have a sexually transmitted infection (STI) and to have been younger at sexual initiation (Cáceres, Vanoss Marín, and Sid Hudes 2000).

A subgroup of youths that is particularly vulnerable to HIV infection is street children (Inciardi and Surratt 1998). An estimated 40 million children, mostly boys, live on the streets of Latin America; both boys and girls frequently survive by sex work, and drug use in this population is high. This group does not have access to, or does not use, mainstream health services. They are focused on short-term survival, and the dangers of HIV/AIDS seem remote and abstract to them. They are often targets of local vigilantes, gangs, and police (Inciardi and Surratt 1998). Projects that have successfully increased risk-reduction behaviors among street children required intense efforts over a long time to achieve results (Adams 2000), and there is a great need for additional work in this area.

Injecting drug use, particularly of cocaine, is an important route of HIV transmission in parts of South America, especially countries in the Southern Cone, Brazil, and Colombia. Access to clean needles and syringes is limited, and sharing of "works" used to inject drugs is common. In addition to the risk of HIV transmission associated with injecting drug use, IDUs may exchange sex for drugs or money, putting them at risk for sexual acquisition of HIV.

CSWs are also at high risk of acquiring and transmitting HIV. Their clients frequently do not use condoms, and sex workers often do not insist on their use because they underestimate the risk of infection, do not have access to condoms, or stand to earn more money by providing unprotected sex (Celantono and others 2000; Grande 2000). In some countries, sex workers are required to register and undergo periodic HIV testing. However, this is not an effective prevention strategy, as it tends to drive sex workers at highest risk underground; sentinel studies, STI surveillance, and condom use studies should be pursued to shed light on this marginalized group (Ecuador 2000). Clients of CSWs act as a bridge between high-risk groups and the general population. This is especially true of men who have sex with male sex workers and are married or have sex with other female partners.

Homosexual behavior is common in Latin America and accounts for a substantial amount of HIV transmission. HIV/AIDS has been concentrated primarily among MSM in Mexico, Costa Rica, and many of the South American countries. Anal intercourse between men and women is also common in Latin America. However, heterosexual anal intercourse is rarely mentioned specifically as a behavior that carries high risk for HIV transmission. Many people are unaware that HIV can be passed this way, and reports of condom use during heterosexual anal intercourse are consistently lower than during vaginal intercourse (Halperin 1998, 1999).

High rates of STIs are documented in some countries and suspected in others. The estimated annual incidence of STIs among 15- to 49-year-olds in Latin America is around 13 percent (PAHO 2001b); table 1.2 lists statistics related to STIs by country or subregion. A person with an STI is at greater risk of HIV infection, both behaviorally and biologically. Since HIV is sexually transmitted, the unsafe sex practices that cause an STI could permit infection with HIV, and the infection itself causes changes in the urogenital tract that can facilitate HIV's entry into cells.

TB is a major problem in Latin America, and the HIV epidemic has exacerbated it. Thirty to 50 percent of adults in Latin America are believed to have latent TB (Zacarías and others 1994), which often takes the opportunity of decreased immunity to awaken. Three to 5 percent of all active TB cases in Latin America are attributed to HIV infection, and 20 percent of PLWHA are believed to have active TB (Zacarías and others 1994). Therefore, increased detection, prevention, and treatment efforts are crucial (*HIV and AIDS in the Americas* 2001; Zacarías and others 1994).

Medications can help reduce the impact of opportunistic infections in PLWHA. Easily obtained, affordable drugs such as antibiotics can prevent infection with common disease-causing organisms. Peru has reported that provision of these drugs has substantially lowered morbidity and mortality from opportunistic infections (Peru 2001). Antiretroviral therapy, which directly inhibits proliferation of HIV, can strengthen the immune system, prolonging lives and significantly improving quality of life. In addition to TB and the opportunistic

Table 1.2. Incidence of Curable Sexually Transmitted Infections, Prevalence of HIV/AIDS, and Incidence of AIDS by Country or Subregion, 1997 and 1999

INDICATOR	MEXICO	CENTRAL AMERICA	BRAZIL	ANDEAN REGION	SOUTHERN CONE
Estimated number of new cases of curable STIs, 1997	6,948,000	2,248,000	12,239,000	8,895,000	3,834,000
Syphilis	538,000	173,000	948,000	795,000	165,000
Gonorrhea	1,399,000	435,000	2,465,000	1,487,000	800,000
Chlamydia	1,681,000	550,000	2,961,000	2,212,000	962,000
Estimated STI incidence in 15- to 49-year-olds, 1997 (per 1,000)	134	130	131	152	126
Estimated number of people living with HIV/AIDS, 1999	150,000	196,900	540,000	204,200	154,000
Estimated HIV/AIDS prevalence in 15- to 49-year-olds, 1999	0.3%	1.1%	0.6%	0.3%	0.5%
Reported new cases of AIDS, 1999	4,372	3,166	18,288	1,727	2,140
Reported AIDS incidence in 15- to 49-year-olds, 1999 (per 1,000,000)	84	183	195	30	70

Note: STI = sexually transmitted infection.
Source: PAHO 2001a.

infections that are common in people living with AIDS in industrial countries, tropical diseases caused by parasites endemic to the region are also a serious concern (Cahn and others 2000).

Several Latin American countries, most notably Brazil, have begun providing antiretroviral drugs to PLWHA at no cost to the patient and without reducing prevention activities. However, preliminary results of a study sponsored by the Regional Initiative on AIDS for Latin America and the Caribbean indicate that most HIV/AIDS budgets in Latin America are directed toward curative services, to the neglect of preventive efforts (Izazola-Licea and others 1998). Antiretroviral therapy accounts for most of these expenditures, although it currently reaches only a fraction of those who need it. Rather than shift funds away from prevention, additional funds should be allocated for treatment. If the proper regimen of antiretroviral therapy is taken on the right schedule, levels of HIV in the blood of an infected person can be reduced to the point that he or she is far less likely to transmit the virus, even during unprotected sex. Moreover, the potential benefits in decreased morbidity and mortality, greater economic productivity, and parenting of children could be substantial.

Mexico

In Mexico, the trend in AIDS incidence has recently leveled off somewhat, with a shift in affected populations toward IDUs and women. However, the epidemic is still largely concentrated in MSM (figure 1.1). Among 25- to 44-year-olds, AIDS is the third most common cause of death in males and the seventh in females (*HIV and AIDS in the Americas* 2001).

A study of over 7,500 MSM between 1991 and 1997 found that more than 15 percent were HIV positive (*HIV and AIDS in the Americas* 2001; UNAIDS 2000p). Eighty-five percent of bisexual Mexican men never used condoms during anal sex with their female partners, and 69 percent never used them during vaginal sex.

As of 1994, 0.6 percent of pregnant women were HIV positive (UNAIDS 2000p), but a 1996–98 study found only 0.09 percent

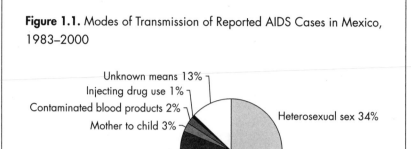

Figure 1.1. Modes of Transmission of Reported AIDS Cases in Mexico, 1983–2000

Unknown means 13%
Injecting drug use 1%
Contaminated blood products 2%
Mother to child 3%

Heterosexual sex 34%

Sex between men 47%

Source: Original survey data.

infected (*HIV and AIDS in the Americas* 2001). Whether this represents a true decline or not is hard to tell. Initially, women were most often infected by contaminated blood products,[2] but this mode of transmission has decreased, and sexual transmission is on the rise (Volkow and others 1998; del Rio Zolezzi and others 1995). Although it is reported that 100 percent of donated blood is screened, historically 7 percent of reported AIDS cases have been attributed to HIV transmission through contaminated blood or blood products (Sepúlveda Amor and others 1995). Box 1.1 discusses blood safety issues in Latin America.

Along with the feminization common to many Latin American countries, there is a phenomenon of "ruralization" of the epidemic in Mexico. The epidemic is growing rapidly among rural populations who have precarious living conditions. Migrant agricultural workers who acquire HIV in the United States may infect their partners after returning to their home communities (Organista and others 1997). As of mid-1994, 25 percent of rural AIDS patients had a history of temporary migration to the United States, as opposed to 6 percent

Box 1.1. Blood Safety

One of the most fundamental steps of HIV prevention is ensuring a safe supply of blood and blood products for medical use. A PAHO report stressed the importance of quality of donors among the first steps toward attaining blood safety (PAHO 2000b). Unpaid volunteer donors are less likely than paid donors to be infected with blood-borne pathogens, including HIV. However, unpaid, volunteer donations are rare in Latin America. Instead, blood is obtained either when a friend or family member "replaces" the blood a patient is given in the hospital or from paid donors.

Latin American governments have recognized that unpaid, voluntary donation is strongly preferred, but the actual administration of blood bank services lags behind this recognition. Most Latin American countries have between 30 and 300 blood banks, except Brazil (1,928), Mexico (597), and Argentina (551) (PAHO 2000b). Blood banks are not centrally administered, and the quality of their services may vary widely even within a single country. Some are administered publicly, some by the Red Cross or other nongovernmental organization (NGO), and others by private companies.

Countries have recognized the need to address the issue of blood safety by creating coherent public policy at the national level. As of 1999, PAHO estimated that 99 percent of all donated blood was screened for HIV. This translates into approximately 50,000 unscreened units per year (PAHO 2000b). A study of 12 Latin American countries in the early 1990s reported that 100 percent of donated blood was screened for HIV in nine countries, making the probability of transfusion-transmitted HIV close to zero in those countries (Schmunis and others 1998). In Colombia, 98.8 percent of donated blood was screened, and the probability of transfusion-transmitted HIV was estimated to be 0.3 per 10,000. In Ecuador, 89.5 percent of donated blood was screened for HIV, with a probability of transfusion-transmitted HIV of 1.0 per 10,000, and in Bolivia, only 36.2 percent of donated blood was screened, with a probability of transfusion-transmitted HIV infection of 0.6 per 10,000. Bolivia has continued to report that only about 40 percent of donated blood is screened for HIV (Schmunis and others 1998).

In southern Brazil, the risk of transfusion-transmitted HIV decreased from 1 per 5,000 in 1991–94 to 1 per 48,777 in 1997–99 (Kupek 2001). However, despite this nearly 10-fold reduction, the risk remains 10 times higher than in industrial countries. Much is yet to be done to secure the Latin American blood supply.

of urban cases (Magis-Rodríguez and others 1995). Only 14 percent of AIDS cases in urban areas occur in women, but in rural areas, women account for 21 percent of cases (Magis-Rodríguez and others 1995).

Studies of female CSWs have reported a low HIV prevalence— below or just at 1.0 percent (Sepúlveda Amor and others 1995; Uribe Zúñiga and others 1995)—while a study of male CSWs found 4.4 percent infected, and several studies conducted by the national program between 1988 and 1997 reported 12.0 percent infected (Mexico 2002). A wider disparity between HIV prevalence in male and female sex workers was found in another study: 12 percent of 104 male CSWs and 0.35 percent of 2,340 female CSWs were positive for HIV (Loo Méndez, Hernández Tepichini, and Terán Toledo 2000). Syphilis rates were similar in the two groups, indicating that they shared behavioral risk factors. High rates of syphilis and other STIs in female sex workers indicate low rates of condom use and high potential for HIV to spread among these workers and their clients (*HIV and AIDS in the Americas* 2001). Condom use among female Mexican CSWs is associated with higher education, greater experience in sex work, and younger age (Loo Méndez, Hernández Tepichini, and Terán Toledo 2000).

A study of teenagers entering high school and university found that among those who were sexually active, 42 percent of males and 36 percent of females had used condoms for their first intercourse. These students had a later age at first intercourse than that reported by other Mexico City teenagers (*HIV and AIDS in the Americas* 2001). A study in Mexico City found limited access to condoms in health clinics and a failure of health care workers to promote condom use for HIV and STI prevention rather than solely as contraceptives (Ortiz-Mondragen and others 2000).

Injecting drug use almost certainly plays a bigger role than reflected in official reports, although even in this population, sex between men is associated with higher risk than injecting drug use alone (PAHO 2000a). Among male IDUs, those who reported sex with men were more than three times as likely as those reporting sex only with women to be HIV positive (Organista and others 1997). Among IDUs in 16 Mexican cities, up to 6 percent of males and 2 percent of females were found to be HIV infected, and 70 percent of IDUs shared works (UNAIDS 2000u).

In the early 1990s, up to 2 percent of TB patients in 17 states were HIV positive (Zwarenstein 2001). High rates of latent TB infection in some parts of Mexico suggest that the number of active TB infections will skyrocket when HIV reaches them (García-García and others 2000). A study in a suburban community in southern Mexico found that nearly a quarter of TB cases were resistant to drugs and that among people with TB, those with HIV were 31 times more likely to die (García-García and others 2000).

Central America

In Central America HIV is overwhelmingly transmitted via heterosexual sex, making it more similar to the countries of the Caribbean than to South America or Mexico (box 1.2). The exception is Costa Rica, where sex between men is the leading mode of transmission (figure 1.2). The three countries with the highest reported HIV prevalence in Latin America (Honduras, Panama, and Guatemala) are in Central America. The situation in this region is grim, and the ability of national health services to address it is inadequate, although Costa Rica is the notable exception. In most Central American countries, like the rest of Latin America, HIV/AIDS care is confined mainly to capital cities and a few other major urban areas, and it competes for scarce resources with other pressing health needs.

Box 1.2. Gender Distribution of Reported AIDS Cases

The HIV/AIDS epidemic in Latin America started primarily in MSM, and in the early years reported AIDS cases were overwhelmingly male. However, there is a general trend in Latin America toward a "feminization" of the HIV/AIDS epidemic as more females are infected, tested, and reported as AIDS cases. While there is likely to be both underdiagnosis and underreporting of AIDS cases, and while reported symptomatic AIDS cases lag up to 10 years behind asymptomatic HIV infections, the changes in the male-to-female AIDS case ratios over time give an indication of the course of the epidemic.

Table 1.3 shows the ratio of reported AIDS cases in males to AIDS cases in females for each of the Latin American countries in 1994 and in 2000 (or 1999, if 2000 data were not available). In every country with available data, with the exception of Chile, the gap in reported AIDS cases between males and females is closing. (In fact, the current figure for Chile is likely to be between 6 and 8, based on previous years' data; at the time the 1999 ratio was calculated, only about one third of the previous years' totals had been reported.)

In Central America, where the epidemic is predominantly heterosexually propagated, the male-to-female ratios for 2000 were low, approaching 1:1 in the case of Honduras. The exception is Costa Rica, where, like Mexico, the epidemic is driven by sex between men.

In the Andean Region and Southern Cone, although ratios have decreased, there is still a higher male-to-female ratio than in Central America. This reflects the greater importance of sex between men in the HIV/AIDS epidemic in South America and also a possible tendency for males to use more injecting drugs.

Cultural factors undoubtedly play a role in the feminization of the HIV/AIDS epidemic in Latin America. For example, females are relatively disempowered in negotiating whether, when, and how to have sex and thus are more vulnerable to infection through involuntary unsafe sex. Males are more likely than females to have multiple partners of either sex and, if infected, may transmit HIV to multiple female partners. In general, females are also less educated than males and may have less access to AIDS information and

(box continued on next page)

Box 1.2. (continued)

Table 1.3. Ratio of Male-to-Female Reported AIDS Cases, 1994 and 2000

COUNTRY	1994	2000
Mexico	6.4	5.6
Central America	2.3	1.8
Guatemala	2.4	1.9
El Salvador	2.8	2.4ᵃ
Honduras	1.7	1.2
Nicaragua	11.7	1.8
Costa Rica	8.6	4.1
Panama	3.3	2.2
Brazil	3.3	1.9
Andean Region	6.5	3.2
Venezuela, R.B. de	7.1	—
Colombia	11.7	5.3
Ecuador	4.3	4.2
Peru	4.6	2.7
Bolivia	3.5	—
Southern Cone	4.1	4.1
Argentina	3.8	3.0
Paraguay	5.8	2.6ᵃ
Uruguay	3.4	2.9ᵃ
Chile	9.6	10.9ᵇ

— Not available.
a. 1999 data.
b. 5.82 in 1999.
Source: Data as of December 2000 from PAHO 2001a.

prevention messages. Adolescent girls are at especially high risk because they are more likely than their male age-mates to be involved with older partners who may transmit HIV to them. The balance of power in such partnerships favors the male; youth, inexperience, and economic inequality are compounded by traditional *machista* values to make women more vulnerable to sexual exploitation and behaviors that put them at higher risk for AIDS and other STIs. Fortunately, education and empowerment programs have had some success in changing the attitudes and practices of both men and women, although widespread social change will take years.

Figure 1.2. Modes of Transmission of Reported AIDS Cases in Central America, 1983–2000

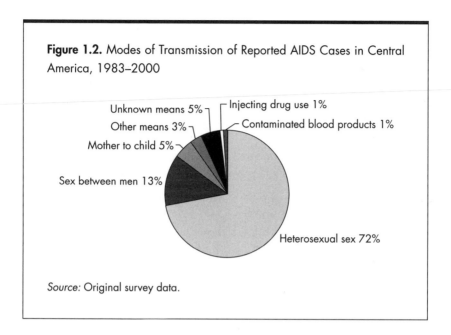

Unknown means 5%
Other means 3%
Mother to child 5%
Sex between men 13%
Injecting drug use 1%
Contaminated blood products 1%
Heterosexual sex 72%

Source: Original survey data.

Guatemala

In Guatemala, the HIV/AIDS epidemic appears to be growing rapidly. It is concentrated in urban areas, especially those along the Pan-American and International Pacific Highways (Guatemala 1999, 2000). The percentage of cases due to heterosexual transmission is unusually high, even when compared with other Central American countries. In the absence of any sentinel studies of HIV prevalence in Guatemalan MSM or IDUs, it is difficult to assess whether this proportion is accurate or whether it reflects underreporting of homosexual behavior.

HIV rates greater than 1 percent have been reported among pregnant women in urban lowland areas (UNAIDS 2000m), although a single study conducted in the highlands suggests HIV was still absent among pregnant women and CSWs as of 1999 (PAHO 2001; UNAIDS 2000m). CSWs in Guatemala City and Puerto Barrios had HIV levels of 5 percent and 11 percent, respectively (*HIV and AIDS in the Americas* 2001; UNAIDS 2000m).

Only 8 percent of female respondents to a 1997 demographic health survey reported ever having used a condom, but another study found that 15 percent of women reported using condoms with their regular partners, and 26 percent used them with other partners (UNAIDS 2000m). Men in the latter study were more likely to report using condoms, with about 35 percent using them with both regular and non-regular partners.

AIDS patients accounted for about 5 percent of hospitalizations in Guatemala (UNAIDS 2000m), and as many as half did not know their infection status before arriving at the hospital. About half of AIDS patients at one hospital in 1998 and 1999 were coinfected with other STIs, which indicates that high-risk sexual behavior continued after HIV infection (UNAIDS 2000m) and the onset of AIDS and that education about safer sex is needed.

A clinic in Guatemala City that does 60 percent of HIV tests in Guatemala found that people who lived farther from the clinic were less likely to return for their results. Only 60 percent of those tested returned; adoption of a rapid test protocol improved the return rate (Samayoa and others 2000).

In one Guatemalan hospital, the percentage of people hospitalized for TB who also tested positive for HIV rose from 1 percent in 1991 to 9.3 percent in 1998 (UNAIDS 2000m). A law mandating testing of donated blood is on the books but has yet to be fully implemented (UNAIDS 2000m).

El Salvador

As in Guatemala, the number of people living with HIV/AIDS in El Salvador continues to rise. The total number of people infected from the start of the epidemic to the end of 1999 was estimated to be between 25,000 and 50,000 (El Salvador 2001). Through 2000, 3,481 cases were reported; 80 percent of reported cases were urban, with 75 percent of those reported from San Salvador (UNAIDS 2000j).

Surveillance data from El Salvador are fairly sparse. CSWs in San Salvador had HIV rates from 2 percent to 7 percent, and one study reported that 6 percent of STI clinic patients were infected with HIV. By contrast, fewer than 2 percent of IDUs tested were HIV positive (UNAIDS 2000j). Percentages of seropositive pregnant women ranged from 0 percent to 1 percent, and 0.15 percent of blood donors tested from 1996 to 1997 had HIV (UNAIDS 2000j). The government has estimated that the average time between HIV infection and onset of AIDS is five to seven years and that 23 years of productive life are lost for each infection (UNAIDS 2000j). Little information on preventive behavior is available, although at least 20 percent of adolescents are estimated to be sexually active. About 3 percent of Salvadoran TB patients are HIV positive.

Honduras

Honduras has the highest prevalence of HIV in all of Latin America, excluding the Caribbean. Although it accounts for just 17 percent of Central America's population, Honduras has reported over 11,000 cases, or 60 percent of Central America's HIV/AIDS cases. The high rates may be due in part to better surveillance. HIV/AIDS is the second leading cause of hospitalization and death in Honduras, after injuries due to violence. AIDS has been the leading cause of death in women of childbearing age since 1997. Although it has the lowest per capita income of any country in Central America, Honduras was the first to implement national surveillance and to provide free HIV testing for all (Honduras 1999).

HIV prevalence is highest in the cities of San Pedro Sula and Tegucigalpa, among the Afro-Carib Garífunas on the Caribbean coast, and along the central corridor between Tegucigalpa and the coast. Ruralization of the epidemic is suspected, but data documenting this are not available (UNAIDS 2000o).

Honduras has the lowest male-to-female ratio of people living with HIV/AIDS in all of Latin America, approaching 1:1. Nationwide, between 1990 and 1998, 1.4 percent of pregnant women were infected with HIV (Cáceres, Vanoss Marín, and Sid Hudes 2000);

2 percent to 5 percent of prenatal clinic patients in San Pedro Sula were infected (UNAIDS 2000w).

In 1997, military recruits were reported to have an HIV prevalence of 6.8 percent, not far behind MSM (8 percent) (*HIV and AIDS in the Americas* 2001). As many as 21 percent of CSWs have tested positive for HIV (*HIV and AIDS in the Americas* 2001; UNAIDS 2000w), but a 1998 study suggests that the true rate among urban CSWs is about 10 percent (UNAIDS 2000o). Preliminary results of a study of female CSWs in Tegucigalpa and San Pedro Sula found 7.7 percent HIV positive, with new cases appearing at a rate of 3.2 percent per year in Tegucigalpa and 0.8 percent per year in San Pedro Sula (Soto and others 2000).

Nearly 7 percent of a population of mostly male prisoners were HIV positive, compared with 0.5 percent of a sample of males more closely resembling the general population. High-risk sexual behavior was common among truck drivers studied in four cities, but those who had sex with other men had six times the risk of HIV infection as those who reported sex exclusively with women (UNAIDS 2000w). Forty percent of these truck drivers said they never used a condom with a CSW, and over 60 percent never used a condom when having sex with domestic workers. Domestic workers appear to be at particular risk of having unwanted unprotected sex: Nearly 70 percent of a sample of Honduran night watchmen reported sex with domestic workers, and only 4 percent always used a condom in this situation (*HIV and AIDS in the Americas* 2001). Injecting drug use is reported to be low in Honduras (UNAIDS 2000o).

Sexually transmitted infections are common in Honduras, and condom use in risky sexual encounters is variable. Garífunas have HIV infection rates six times the national average, with 8.2 percent of men and 8.5 percent of women infected. Sixteen percent of Garífunas in their 20s were HIV positive, despite high levels of knowledge about HIV transmission and prevention (see box 1.3).

About 3 percent of Honduran TB patients are coinfected with HIV, and about 23 percent of AIDS patients have TB (UNAIDS 2000o).

Box 1.3. Special Considerations for Indigenous Populations

Latin American populations and cultures are amazingly diverse, comprising many indigenous groups and some African-Caribbean populations, as well as the dominant *mestizo* or *criollo* population. The risk for, prevalence of, and level of knowledge about HIV/AIDS are understudied in many of these groups. In general, indigenous populations suffer from excess morbidity and mortality related to poverty. For example, over 70 percent of 179 Native Americans surveyed in the Peruvian Amazon had no access to a physician. Use of prenatal services was low in this group. In Chiapas, Mexico, indigenous people were among those most likely to present with advanced TB or not to seek treatment at all (Sánchez Pérez and Halperin Frisch 1997).

Many indigenous populations have so far been spared from HIV/AIDS because of their geographic and cultural isolation, but available data on traditional STIs and other human viral and retroviral infections make it clear that behavioral risk factors for HIV transmission exist in these populations. Thus, there is a need for appropriate HIV/AIDS services targeted to these groups.

In a few cases, indigenous or minority populations have higher rates of HIV infection than the general population. For instance, the Garífunas along the Atlantic coast of Honduras have rates of HIV infection that are six times higher than the general Honduran population, despite the fact that their knowledge of risk factors for HIV and preventive measures are reportedly very high. A study in El Salvador pointed out that people may correctly identify HIV risks when asked but may also have incorrect knowledge about HIV risk. If incorrect ideas are given the same weight as correct ones, perceptions of personal risk and adoption of preventive behaviors may not be appropriate. These findings may account for some of the discrepancy between knowledge and practice (London and Robles 2000).

For the most part, the indigenous peoples of the Central American and Andean highlands have very low rates of HIV infection. Guatemala is a case in point: HIV infection in pregnant women

(*box continued on next page*)

Box 1.3. (continued)

exceeds 1 percent in some urban lowland areas but is virtually absent in the highlands, which are predominantly populated by Mayan Indians. A study found that only 47 percent of 210 rural Mayan women had heard of AIDS; 81 percent of these knew that a woman could be infected, and 79 percent did not know where to buy condoms. A Guatemalan NGO is working to indirectly increase HIV/AIDS awareness in these communities by providing HIV/AIDS education to young men, many of whom are Mayan, during their obligatory military service (Cano Flores and Chávez Espina 2000).

HTLV-1 and HTLV-2, human retroviruses related to HIV, are endemic among native American groups in South America (Medeot and others 1999). The presence and transmission of these viruses, which are spread by the same routes as HIV, indicate the potential for HIV to spread if it were to gain a foothold. The archaeological record indicates that HTLV-1 and HTLV-2 have been in those populations for millennia, probably carried from Asia by the first settlers of the Americas (Cartier, Araya, and others 1993; Cartier, Tajima, and others 1993). Likewise, hepatitis B and hepatitis D viruses are endemic and have caused outbreaks among Native Americans in northern South America and the Amazon Basin (Echevarría, Blitz-Dorfman, and Pujot 1996; León and others 1999; Manock and others 2000; Sonoda and others 2000). A study of more than 1,000 members of 18 different American Indian tribes in Colombia found no HIV infections, although other retroviruses were found in this group (Duenas-Barajas and others 1993). Among 276 female and 94 male Quechua Indians in Cuzco and Quillabamba, Peru, only one was HIV positive, but 5 percent were infected with HTLV-I (Zurita and others 1997). The one person infected with HIV was a man who had sex with men and was probably infected outside the community. HIV had not been introduced among the heterosexual population, but infection with HTLV-I was associated with risky sexual behaviors and a history of STIs. In a study in Manaus, in northeastern Brazil, 31 indigenous people were infected with a strain of HIV that was linked to the urban HIV epidemic in southeastern Brazil (Vicente and others 2000). The trafficking of cocaine in remote regions and the associated rise in drug-related HIV infection suggest that all but the most isolated groups may soon be at risk of HIV infection.

Nicaragua

Nicaragua was sheltered from the early years of the HIV/AIDS epidemic by the Contra war in the 1980s, the U.S.-led embargo, low rates of injecting drug use, and no importation of blood products before the ousting of the Sandinistas in 1990 (Low and others 1993). As of September 1999, 476 HIV/AIDS cases, of whom 209 had AIDS, had been identified in Nicaragua (Nicaragua 2000). Over half of all reported cases in Nicaragua are concentrated in Managua. Surveillance data on HIV levels in pregnant women are not available. A study of MSM in Managua found 2 percent HIV positive, and another of CSWs in Managua in 1990–91 reported a seroprevalence of 1 percent (UNAIDS 2000q). Blood donors had HIV prevalence rates of 0.05–0.07 percent.

STIs, especially gonorrhea and syphilis, are reported to be "out of control" in Nicaragua, but specific data on prevalence are unavailable. Knowledge of proper condom use is low. An intervention in Managua succeeded in increasing condom use somewhat, from 9 percent to 16 percent in women and from 31 percent to 41 percent in men (Pauw and others 1996). In a study in Managua hotels used for commercial and noncommercial sexual rendezvous, condom use in commercial encounters was 60 percent and in noncommercial encounters 20 percent (Egger and others 2000).

Prevention messages are primarily delivered in Spanish and aimed at the mestizo population, neglecting the English-speaking indigenous population on the Atlantic coast. However, condom use doubled from 35 percent to 71 percent between 1991 and 1997 among Atlantic coast men who had sex with more than one partner in the year prior to the survey (*HIV and AIDS in the Americas* 2001).

Costa Rica

Costa Rica is unique among Central American nations in the predominance of MSM among people living with HIV/AIDS. The prevalence of HIV in MSM has been reported to be between 10 percent and 16 percent (UNAIDS 2000w). Studies of pregnant women in Costa Rica as late as 1997 found HIV in 0.5 percent or less

(UNAIDS 2000h). Between 1 percent and 4 percent of STI clinic patients in San Jose from 1990 to 1994 were infected with HIV, and seropositivity in CSWs tested between 1989 and 1997 ranged from 0.1 percent to 2.0 percent (UNAIDS 2000h). HIV/AIDS infections are concentrated in urban zones.

Costa Rica is also unique in that its social security system covers all citizens and provides comprehensive HIV/AIDS care. CD4 cell counts, viral load testing, medications to treat TB and other opportunistic infections, and antiretroviral drugs are all available (Wheeler and others 2001). A decrease in progression to AIDS and death from AIDS has been reported among Costa Ricans receiving antiretroviral therapy.

Literacy is extremely high in Costa Rica, and the population is well informed about HIV/AIDS prevention (UNAIDS 2000h). In 1995 WHO estimated that 96 percent of people had access to condoms, and PAHO reported that for men, approximately 75 percent of 15- to 19-year-olds, 55 percent of 20- to 29-year-olds, 47 percent of 30- to 39-year-olds, and 37 percent of 40- to 49-year-olds used condoms with casual partners in 2000 (*HIV and AIDS in the Americas* 2001). In another study, 55 percent of males and 42 percent of females reported using a condom for their last risky intercourse (UNAIDS 2000h).

Panama

Panama has the second-highest rate of HIV/AIDS in Central America after Honduras. Very few data are available on HIV prevalence in specific high-risk groups in Panama. HIV prevalence in both pregnant women and CSWs has been reported to be as high as 0.9 percent in major urban areas (*HIV and AIDS in the Americas* 2001; UNAIDS 2000r); no information on HIV among MSM or IDUs is available. A 1991 study may give a more accurate glimpse of the true penetration of HIV into Panama's population; 5.8 percent of military recruits were found to be infected with HIV (Panama 1999). Indications are that both HIV and traditional STIs like gonorrhea are increasing in Panama (Panama 1999).

Brazil

UNAIDS, WHO, and PAHO have estimated that the number of PLWHA in Brazil at the end of 1999 was 540,000 (*HIV and AIDS in the Americas* 2001). The government's unique and ambitious program to provide affordable, locally produced antiretroviral therapy means that this number will continue to grow as people with AIDS live longer, despite the leveling off of new cases. One clinic in São Paulo reported a reduction in AIDS-related mortality from 42.2 per 100 in 1996, when antiretroviral therapy was introduced, to 15.9 per 100 in 1999 (Kalichman and others 2000). The negative side of widespread antiretroviral use is that resistance to these drugs is appearing in some people infected with HIV, meaning that the drugs are no longer effective in fighting the virus. Nearly a fifth of all reported AIDS cases in Brazil are not assigned to an exposure category; the remainder are nearly evenly divided between sex between men and heterosexual sex, with injecting drug use accounting for nearly 20 percent of the total cases of AIDS (UNAIDS 2000d, see figure 1.3).

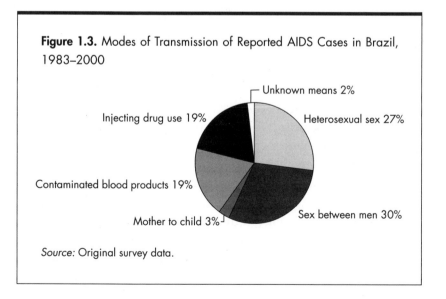

Figure 1.3. Modes of Transmission of Reported AIDS Cases in Brazil, 1983–2000

Unknown means 2%

Heterosexual sex 27%

Injecting drug use 19%

Contaminated blood products 19%

Mother to child 3%

Sex between men 30%

Source: Original survey data.

The HIV/AIDS epidemic is most severe in the cities of the south and southeast. Sixty percent of Brazilians living with HIV/AIDS are in Rio de Janeiro and São Paulo. While sex between men was initially the major mode of transmission, heterosexual transmission has been the dominant mode of transmission since the mid-1990s. This transition may be due in part to the relative popularity of anal intercourse among heterosexuals. Fifty to 60 percent of women in general surveys, and 32–41 percent of HIV-negative female partners of HIV-positive men, reported practicing anal intercourse. Reported condom use in heterosexual anal intercourse is consistently less than in vaginal intercourse (Halperin 1998, 1999).

At the same time, condom use in general has taken off in Brazil, with sales more than quadrupling between 1993 and 1999 (UNAIDS 2000w). In Rio de Janeiro, men who had anal sex with men increased condom use from 34 percent in 1989 to 69 percent in 1995 (UNAIDS 2000w). A study of 16- to 25-year-olds reported that 87 percent used condoms with casual partners, while another study in 1999 found that close to half of young men reported having used a condom for their first sex act, with condom use higher among more educated men (UNAIDS 2000w; Kerr-Pontes and others 1999). Condom use is not universal; in areas where the HIV epidemic is just picking up, such as Fortaleza in the northeast, it is less common (UNAIDS 2000w; Kerr-Pontes and others 1999). Researchers visiting health centers in São Paulo found inadequate condom supplies (Barboza and others 2000), possibly a consequence of the concentration of resources on treatment rather than prevention.

In northeastern Brazil, HIV infection has remained concentrated among MSM, although a growing number of women are infected by sex with these men. Nationwide, the number of HIV infections among MSM is estimated to be increasing by 1.5–3 percent per year (Cáceres and Chequer 2000).

HIV prevalence among pregnant 13- to 24-year-olds in the country as a whole was 0.4 percent in 1998, but prevalence in the same age group in the southeast was 1.7 percent in 1997. Among women delivering at a facility for high-risk pregnancies in São Paulo, 1.5 percent were HIV positive. In Vitória, 0.6 percent of 600 pregnant women were HIV positive (Miranda, Alves, and others 2000), but the highest prevalence among pregnant females was in the city of Porto Alegre in Rio Grande do Sul, where HIV prevalence in 1996–97 was 2.6–3.3 percent (Bergenstrom and Sherr 2000). This number may be somewhat inflated because some providers reported testing for HIV selectively, despite a policy that HIV testing should be offered to *all* pregnant women.

HIV/AIDS is affecting younger and poorer segments of Brazil's population, but the epidemic is not limited to youths. A study of AIDS in the state of Rio found that 3 percent of people living with HIV/AIDS were over 60 years old (Sanches and others 2000). As survival increases because of treatment with antiretroviral drugs, more people with AIDS can be expected to live longer.

Injecting drug use has emerged as a major factor in the HIV/AIDS epidemic in Brazil. IDUs in Santos reported that their drug-related risk behavior was decreasing more quickly than their sex-related risk behavior (Bueno and others 2000). Likewise, one-third of IDUs in Rio reported sharing needles, but twice that number (63 percent) said they never used condoms with casual sex partners, and one third had traded sex for drugs (UNAIDS 2000w). IDUs with AIDS were at higher risk for TB than MSM with AIDS (Belo and others 2000). A small study of IDUs in Porto Alegre and Rio found a higher HIV prevalence in Porto Alegre, where higher incomes allowed IDUs to inject more frequently (Surratt 2000). Needle exchange programs have recently been approved in Brazil (UNAIDS 2000w), which hopefully will increase access to clean needles and decrease transmission among IDUs.

Brazil has 7–8 million street children between the ages of 5 and 18 who are at high risk for HIV through drug use and unprotected sex (Inciardi and Surratt 1998). Most drugs used by these children are smoked or inhaled, but in a study in Belo Horizonte, 10 percent admitted to injecting drugs. Another study, by an NGO working with street children in Belo Horizonte over the course of 10 years, found that exchanging sex for money, not using condoms, injecting drugs, and smoking crack were associated with HIV (Adams 2000).

Youths in prisons, a population that overlaps with street children, are also at high risk for HIV. HIV prevalence in the general prison population in Brazil is between 12 percent and 17 percent. Among 121 adult female prisoners in Vitória, 10 percent were HIV positive, and many had other STIs (Miranda, Vargas, and others 2000). A 1998 study found that 18 percent of CSWs in São Paulo were infected and that 3.7 percent of men and 1.2 percent of women attending STI clinics were HIV positive (UNAIDS 2000d).

Andean Region

There are signs that the epidemic in the Andean region is growing. There is strong evidence of risky sexual behavior; this region has the highest estimated incidence of STI infection (15 percent) in all of Latin America (PAHO 2001b), which indicates that the HIV/AIDS epidemic may be worse than the epidemiological surveillance systems detect. Over 40 percent of reported AIDS cases are attributed to sex between men (box 1.4), with a nearly equal number attributed to heterosexual sex. Injecting drug use makes a negligible contribution; about 15 percent of cases with unknown sources of exposure may actually be associated with injecting drug use (figure 1.4).

Information from sentinel surveillance and seroprevalence and behavioral studies is limited. Underreporting of HIV/AIDS is probably substantial in this region; resources are scarce and surveillance systems weak in the República Bolivariana de Venezuela, Ecuador, and Bolivia.

República Bolivariana de Venezuela

The República Bolivariana de Venezuela has the highest estimated HIV prevalence in the Andean region, but without data on high-risk groups, the epidemic is classified as low level. Over 8,000 AIDS cases were registered by the Ministry of Health and Social Development (Venezuela 2001), and PAHO, WHO, and UNAIDS estimated that about 62,000 people were living with HIV/AIDS at the end of 1999.

Box 1.4. Sex between Men and HIV/AIDS in Latin America

As of the end of 2000, sex between men accounted for a third of all reported AIDS cases in Latin America. Because of the particular vulnerability of MSM to HIV infection as a consequence of behaviors such as unprotected anal intercourse, relations with multiple partners, and commercial sex work, it is important to understand the dynamics of behavior in this heterogeneous group.

Male homosexual behavior is generally clandestine and occurs on the margins, such as late at night in discos or bars outside the mainstream. Separate gay-identified communities, such as those found in the United States in San Francisco or New York, are virtually unknown in Latin America. As long as it is not explicitly discussed, homosexual behavior is tacitly accepted or ignored by family members and social contacts. For instance, in Nicaragua, MSM are integrated into family and neighborhood life and are described as being "known about" rather than "recognized" (Adam 1993). MSM who have a more public gay identity are frequently the targets of hostility and violence, and social and cultural stigma remains associated with homosexuality. Gay-identified men in Guatemala City reported being profoundly marginalized; they felt that they were disenfranchised and had no recourse if they were abused (Rodríguez and others 2000).

The silence and marginalization that MSM in Latin America endure contribute to their susceptibility to HIV infection. With little sense of community among MSM and few activist groups, it is difficult to spread the AIDS prevention message and create a culture of safe sex practice. In Lima, Peru, MSM reported that they had insufficient information about AIDS and that safer sex was inconsistently practiced, especially in commercial sex (Zuloaga Posada, Soto Vélez, and Jaramillo Vélez 1995). Likewise, among MSM in Fortaleza, Brazil, 43 percent did not have the fundamental information needed to protect themselves from HIV. Only half had ever been tested, and 44 percent reported engaging in unprotected anal sex. This differs from the situation among MSM in southern Brazil,

(box continued on next page)

Box 1.4. *(continued)*

where sexual and cultural norms are more relaxed and gay culture is described as "out of the closet for good" (Klein 1999).

To control the HIV/AIDS epidemic in Latin America, and especially in those countries where sex between men is the dominant mode of transmission (Mexico, Costa Rica, and much of South America), it is imperative that health care and prevention messages be provided to MSM in safe, respectful contexts. While Latin American societies still have a long way to go in granting recognition and basic rights to MSM, advances are being made.

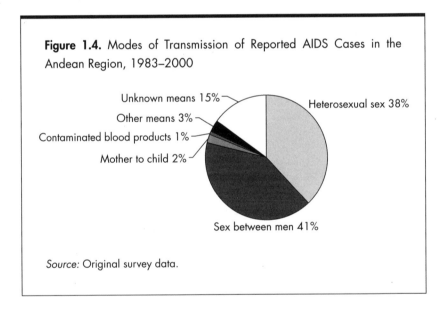

Figure 1.4. Modes of Transmission of Reported AIDS Cases in the Andean Region, 1983–2000

Unknown means 15%
Other means 3%
Contaminated blood products 1%
Mother to child 2%
Heterosexual sex 38%
Sex between men 41%

Source: Original survey data.

In 1996, AIDS was the sixth most common cause of death in 25- to 44-year-olds. HIV rates are higher on Margarita Island and Venezuela's other Caribbean islands than on the mainland. Among residents of mining communities, prevalence was 1 percent (*HIV and AIDS in the Americas* 2001). Very little information about the

HIV/AIDS epidemic in Venezuela is available, but it appears to be increasing in tourist, industrial, and mining areas (Venezuela 2001).

Surveys of pregnant women in Venezuela in 1996 found no HIV infections, and prevalence in CSWs in Caracas has ranged from 0 percent to 6 percent (UNAIDS 2000z). Of 400 prisoners tested in 1996, 2.5 percent were HIV positive (*HIV and AIDS in the Americas* 2001). These data suggest that the HIV epidemic in Venezuela is more advanced than is indicated by official statistics.

Colombia

In Colombia, sex between men is the primary mode of transmission in the highlands, and heterosexual transmission plays a larger role in the Atlantic Coast region, Orinoquia, and the Amazon region.

Studies of Colombian CSWs have found an HIV prevalence in the range of 0.2 percent to 0.9 percent, but among one sample of more than 100 male and female teenage sex workers, 11 percent were HIV positive. Nearly 20 percent of the group also had syphilis. A 1991 survey of university students found that 17 percent of males and 3 percent of females had a history of an STI (Zuloaga Posada, Soto Vélez, and Jaramillo Vélez, 1995), and a 1999 study of male and female STI clinic patients found 1.1 percent HIV positive (*HIV and AIDS in the Americas* 2001); four out of 12 departments reported prevalence rates of 2 percent or more among STI clinic patients. Between 0.1 percent and 0.7 percent of pregnant women in Colombia have been reported to be HIV positive (*HIV and AIDS in the Americas* 2001).

MSM are the group with the highest reported HIV prevalence in Colombia, with 18 percent of MSM tested in Bogotá in 1999 positive for the virus (*HIV and AIDS in the Americas* 2001). Interestingly, a study from Bogotá published in 2001 reported that heterosexuals were significantly more likely than homosexuals to engage in risky sexual behavior. Only 2 percent of the 553 men in the study knew their HIV serostatus, and only 20 percent of those who practiced anal sex and 5 percent of those who had sex with women during menses reported consistent condom use (*HIV and AIDS in the Americas* 2001).

In contrast to the 2001 study, an earlier survey reported higher condom use. Fifty-five percent of men surveyed claimed they always used a condom with casual anal sex partners, and in another survey of men with no steady partner, 75 percent reported having used a condom in their last sex act. Condom use among women was much lower: The 2000 demographic and health survey reported that only 19 percent of women surveyed had ever used a condom (UNAIDS 2000f). In Cúcuta, a region where heterosexual transmission dominates, a behavioral intervention among 93 women increased condom use, especially during anal sex (García and others 2000). In another study, only 6 percent of 700 women representative of the general population, but 67 percent of 412 female CSWs, reported consistent condom use. Over half the respondents in both groups were unaware of the increased risk of HIV transmission associated with sex during menses (Miguez-Burbano and others 2000). Six percent to 9 percent of TB patients tested in the mid-1990s were HIV positive (*HIV and AIDS in the Americas* 2001).

Injecting drug use, although not reported in current official statistics, probably accounts for a substantial proportion of AIDS cases. Eight years ago, official statistics reported IDU prevalence at 0.1 percent.

Ecuador

Data on the current status of the HIV/AIDS epidemic in Ecuador are very scarce. A document generated internally reported a total of 2,668 HIV/AIDS cases from 1984 to 1999, of which 1,457 had progressed to AIDS at the time of report (Ecuador 2000). Three-quarters of Ecuador's AIDS cases have been reported from the province of Guayas, largely because Guayas is the site of the infectious disease hospital, where many AIDS cases are first diagnosed after patients make their way there for treatment (Ecuador 2000).

The proportion of females infected with HIV is increasing in Ecuador, although the prevalence of HIV among pregnant women in 2001 was reported to be just 0.05 percent. An earlier study from Guayaquil reported that 0.3 percent of pregnant women were HIV positive (UNAIDS 2000i). No estimates of HIV prevalence among MSM, IDUs, or CSWs were found. A survey of CSWs found that 80 percent had an STI, and a sharp increase in STIs among 14- to 19-year-olds has been reported. Studies of STI clinic patients in Quito in 1992 found 0.5 percent HIV positive, and a study in Guayaquil in 1993 found 3.5 percent HIV positive (*HIV and AIDS in the Americas* 2001). In 2000, 0.26 percent of blood donors were infected (Ecuador 2000).

In a study of 870 secondary school students at four schools in Quito and four schools in the Amazon region, sexual activity was reported by 41 percent of urban and 52 percent of rural respondents. Of those sexually active, 50 percent never used condoms, and 70 percent had not used a condom in their last risky intercourse (Park and others 2000). Condom supplies are reported to be low. An assessment of Ecuador's epidemiological surveillance system concluded that HIV/AIDS surveillance and prevention activities have decreased in relation to an increase in dengue and malaria control activities following a World Bank grant focused on these mosquito-borne diseases (Ecuador 2000).

Peru

As of December 2000, over 11,000 HIV/AIDS cases were reported in Peru. Another 75,000 people are believed to be HIV positive but have not been tested. In Peru, HIV infection is concentrated among the poor in coastal cities—two-thirds of reported cases are in Lima and the adjoining Callao area (Peru 2001). The highest rates of infection have been reported in MSM, although the proportion of females is increasing. HIV prevalence varies widely by region: In one study, 14 percent of MSM in Lima and 5 percent of MSM in the provinces tested positive for HIV (UNAIDS 2000w). In another study of close to 5,000 MSM conducted in 1998, HIV was detected in 12.2 percent of those in Lima, 14.5 percent in Iquitos, and 7.5 percent in Pucallpa (both cities in the Amazonian region); 2.7 percent to 5.3 percent in coastal cities; and 1.4 percent in the Andean city of Cuzco. In the entire sample, consistent condom use was reported by only 12 percent, and 46 percent of MSM also reported engaging in sex with women. Among transvestites in this sample, HIV prevalence was 35 percent (Jorge and others 2000). A study of MSM in Lima estimated that new cases occurred at the rate of 3.3 per 1,000 per year (Sánchez and others 2000). Other areas with increasing rates of HIV incidence are the northern coastal city of Chiclayo and the Amazon city of Iquitos, where homosexual tourism contributes to the epidemic (Cáceres and Rosasco 1999).

Other high-risk populations had lower HIV prevalence. Nationwide, 0.6 percent to 2.0 percent of CSWs are positive for HIV, although levels as high as 5 percent have been reported in urban areas, and between 1986 and 1990, 10 percent of unlicensed CSWs were HIV positive. Among 100 female CSWs in Lima, regular condom use was reported by 87 percent, although by only 29 percent of those who had a regular partner and used condoms (Celantono and others 2000). Seven percent of STI patients tested in 1995 were HIV positive (Peru 2001).

HIV rates in pregnant women are still well below 1 percent in Lima and lower still in the provinces (Peru 2001). Sentinel surveillance among 15- to 24-year-olds at maternity hospitals in Lima found 0.23–0.58 percent to be HIV positive between 1996 and 1999 (*HIV and AIDS in the Americas* 2001). AIDS cases are increasing in 20- to 24-year-olds, indicating that HIV infection is occurring in teenagers (Peru 2001).

The role of injecting drug use in the Peruvian HIV epidemic is difficult to evaluate, because no data on the prevalence of HIV among IDUs are available after 1990. A nationwide serosurvey conducted between 1986 and 1990 reported that 13 percent of IDUs were HIV positive (McCarthy and others 1996). In 1998, 0.23 percent of blood donors in Peru were infected with HIV (*HIV and AIDS in the Americas* 2001).

STIs are common in Peru, although exact frequencies are hard to come by. In one survey of young adults, more than 10 percent had an STI; in another survey of men in their 20s, 12–16 percent reported STI symptoms in the previous year, but as many as two-thirds sought no treatment (*HIV and AIDS in the Americas* 2001). Positive syphilis serology among pregnant 15- to 24-year-olds in Lima ranged from 8 percent to 17 percent between 1996 and 1998 (UNAIDS 2000t). In the 1986–90 serosurvey, 10 percent of STI clinic patients were HIV positive.

Since 1995, the government has provided drugs to prevent some opportunistic infections associated with HIV/AIDS, resulting in a decrease in those infections (Peru 2001).

Bolivia

Bolivia's risk factors are similar to those of its neighboring countries. UNAIDS, WHO, and PAHO estimates indicate that about 4,200 people were living with HIV/AIDS at the end of 1999 (*HIV and AIDS in the Americas* 2001). As of March 2000, 498 HIV/AIDS cases had been reported, nearly half of which presented with AIDS at the time of report (UNAIDS 2000c). Only 3 percent of identified AIDS patients survive more than three years (Bolivia 2000a), a figure that attests to lack of access and the reluctance of people to seek testing and treatment until late in the course of illness. Virtually all reports of HIV and AIDS in Bolivia come from urban areas, primarily from the central corridor of La Paz, Cochabamba, and Santa Cruz, where there is a lot of traffic and where internal migrants tend to settle (Bolivia 2000b).

Bolivia lacks data on the prevalence of HIV among MSM and IDUs but has good STI surveillance data. Syphilis, primarily detected in prenatal screening programs, has increased over the past decade, and congenital syphilis has increased as well. Rates of gonorrhea, primarily detected in 20- to 29-year-old males, more than doubled between 1984 and 1998 (Bolivia 2000a; ONUSIDA 2000a). Despite high rates of traditional STIs in pregnant women, between 1990 and 1997, no HIV infections were detected in prenatal screening in two Bolivian cities. However, in 1997, 0.5 percent of pregnant women tested in Cochabamba were HIV positive (UNAIDS 2000c). Females are believed to represent a third of those living with HIV/AIDS in Bolivia (Bolivia 2000a).

Among STI clinic patients surveyed in 2000, 0.03 percent were HIV positive. An estimate of 0.3 percent HIV prevalence among

CSWs was obtained from a study in 1998 in which CSWs volunteered to be tested, but this is likely to underestimate the true prevalence, as those most at risk may have been less likely to volunteer for testing. The estimated true prevalence in CSWs is 0.5 percent. An HIV prevention project targeted at female sex workers in La Paz increased reported condom use in this group from 36 percent in 1992 to 73 percent in 1995, with concomitant decreases in STIs diagnosed. In 1995, HIV seroprevalence in this group of about 500 female CSWs was 0.1 percent (Levine and others 1998).

In a 1998 survey, 46 percent of women of childbearing age believed that using a condom prevents AIDS, and 3 percent of women and 19 percent of men reported that they began using condoms as a means of AIDS prevention. In another survey, 65 percent of males and 33 percent of females reported having used a condom during their last risky sex act.

Southern Cone

In the Southern Cone the epidemic is persistently growing in the marginalized populations and spreading to the general population. Argentina has the highest prevalence of HIV infection in South America and one of the highest percentages of infected children, and HIV infections are on the rise. Among reported AIDS cases, injecting drug use plays the largest role, closely followed by sex between men (UNAIDS 2000b). While there is probably a great deal of underreporting, as in the other regions, the Southern Cone has the lowest percentage of cases with an unknown or unclassified mode of transmission (figure 1.5).

HIV infection resulting from injecting drug use is particularly high in Argentina and Uruguay but much less common in Chile, where sex between men is the primary mode of transmission. Very few cases have been reported from Paraguay, and the majority of these infections were heterosexually acquired. However, other data indicate that injecting drug use may play a role in HIV transmission in Paraguay (box 1.5).

Figure 1.5. Modes of Transmission of Reported AIDS Cases in the Southern Cone, 1983–2000

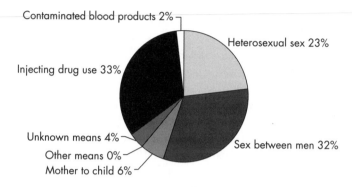

Contaminated blood products 2%

Heterosexual sex 23%

Injecting drug use 33%

Unknown means 4%

Other means 0%

Mother to child 6%

Sex between men 32%

Source: Original survey data.

Box 1.5. Intertwined Epidemics: Injecting Drug Use and HIV

Injecting drug use is especially high in Brazil, Argentina, Uruguay, and Mexico, and it is a growing problem in cocaine-producing countries like Bolivia, Peru, and Colombia. Drug injection increases the risk of infection with HIV through several routes: (1) use of a needle previously used by someone with HIV; (2) exchange of sex, often unprotected, for drugs or for money to buy drugs; and (3) engagement in high-risk behavior while under the influence of drugs.

The drug of choice for IDUs in Latin America is cocaine; heroin use is less frequent, especially in South America (Libonatti and others 1993; Lima and others 1994). People often start by snorting or smoking cocaine and then switch to injecting. In 1996–97, a study of nearly 300 Brazilian cocaine users found that 87 percent started by snorting cocaine; 68 percent later switched to smoking cocaine and 20 percent to injecting. Both smoking and injecting

(*box continued on next page*)

Box 1.5. (*continued*)

were associated with higher dependence than snorting. Younger users and those who started after 1990 were less likely to inject (Dunn and Laranjeira 1999).

Cocaine use poses a greater risk for HIV infection than heroin, because cocaine is often injected many times a day. The high frequency of injection may lead cocaine injectors to neglect safer injection techniques; cocaine can also be a sexual stimulant, and therefore users may be more likely to engage in risky sexual behavior. As early as 1986–87, 47 percent of 99 IDUs in Buenos Aires who had hepatitis were also infected with HIV (Diaz Lestrem and others 1989), and by 1991, more than one quarter of all reported AIDS cases in Brazil and Argentina were transmitted by injecting drug use. The greatest risks for HIV infection among cocaine injectors include injecting more than five times per day, failing to adopt AIDS prevention behaviors, and sex between men (Barbosa de Carvalho and others 1996).

The major trafficking routes from the coca-growing countries are through Brazil, and cities along those routes have twice as many AIDS cases as other Brazilian cities and four times as many AIDS cases among IDUs. In Santos, Brazil, the largest port in Latin America, approximately 2 percent of the population are IDUs (Barbosa de Carvalho and others 1996).

Crack cocaine was introduced to Brazil in 1989, and studies in the Santos metropolitan area showed that crack smoking increased from 11 percent in 1991–92 to 67 percent in 1999 (Ferri and Gossop 1999), while the prevalence of injecting cocaine more than five times per day decreased from 42 percent to 15 percent over the same period (Surratt 2000; Mesquita and others 2001). HIV prevalence also decreased from 63 percent to 42 percent during this period in the absence of any major public health intervention (Ferri and Gossop 1999).

However, the injection-associated HIV epidemic shows no sign of abating in Brazil. HIV is moving into younger age groups and into more impoverished and more rural areas of the country (Surratt and others 2000). Interestingly, HIV is not the only blood-borne infection transmitted by injecting drugs; malaria is being spread to urban areas at the same time that HIV/AIDS is spreading into rural malarial areas along drug trafficking routes. Despite the huge injecting drug use problem, there is little access to treatment. Drug treatment in Brazil is available only through private or religious centers and is too expensive for most drug users.

Without effective treatment options, IDUs are frequently relegated to the criminal justice system. The prison environment has been described as "selectively enriched" with IDUs, as many IDUs have criminal records related to their illegal drug use or drug-related crimes. Indeed, injecting drug use and imprisonment are closely related: In 1993–94, 22 percent of prisoners in a Brazilian prison reported injecting drugs; overall, 16 percent were HIV positive, and 18 percent had syphilis (Burattini and others 2000; Massad and others 1999). Similar data exist for Argentina: In Buenos Aires between 1992 and 1995, nearly 5 percent of imprisoned teens were HIV positive, and in Rosario, 26 percent of youths detained by police injected drugs (Maidagan and others 2000). HIV risk increases with duration of incarceration, since injecting drug use continues in prison (Burattini and others 2000; Massad and others 1999).

There is an urgent need for injecting drug use to be addressed in Latin America from a medical, rather than a law enforcement, standpoint. Drug users come from all segments of society and may provide a bridge by which HIV can cross to the general population. The lack of data from countries outside Brazil and, to a lesser extent, Argentina and Mexico does not imply that other countries are free of injecting drug use. Rather, the clandestine nature of illegal drug use, the marginalization of drug users, and the unwillingness to confront this problem have impeded the collection of basic data on this population at high risk for HIV infection.

Argentina

Ninety percent of AIDS cases in Argentina are reported from urban areas, with Buenos Aires accounting for 36 percent, followed by cities in the southern and western regions (Argentina 2000). In Rosario,

0.5 percent of 11,000 volunteers were HIV positive, with the highest prevalence among 30- to 40-year-olds (Ludo and others 2000). Nationwide, HIV prevalence in pregnant women is estimated to be between 0.6 and 0.7 percent, but rates in major urban areas may be as high as 2 percent (UNAIDS 2000b). The mean age and educational level of women with AIDS were substantially lower than those of men, and one-third of women with AIDS acquired it through injecting drug use (Argentina 2000).

Among 130 maternity patients in Buenos Aires, injecting drug use, irregular condom use, and heterosexual anal intercourse were associated with HIV (Pando and others 2000).

Very high rates of HIV infection in IDUs have been reported, with 46 percent estimated to be HIV positive as of 2000 (Argentina 2000). Three-quarters of IDUs in Buenos Aires reported sharing injection paraphernalia, and efforts to address this problem by improving access to clean needles at pharmacies were reported at the International AIDS Conference in 2000 (Cymerman and others 2000). IDUs living with AIDS are younger, less educated, and more concentrated in Buenos Aires, Rosario, and Cordoba than those who acquired AIDS through other routes (Argentina 2000). Up to one-third have traded sex for drugs (UNAIDS 2000w).

Among 111 detainees in Rosario police stations, 9 percent were HIV positive, and 84 percent did not use condoms, although they knew condoms prevented AIDS. Twenty-six percent were IDUs. Similarly, among teens in correctional facilities in Buenos Aires in 1992–95, 4.6 percent were HIV positive, and HIV infection was highly associated with injecting drug use (Ávila and others 1996).

Data on HIV prevalence in Argentine MSM were not available for this study. Three percent to 8 percent of CSWs tested in the early 1990s were infected (Zapiola and others 1996). Fifteen percent of 200 CSWs in Buenos Aires were HIV positive in one sample, with higher rates among those in saunas or massage houses as opposed to those in hotels or on the streets.

In a sample of 33 CSWs in Rosario, 82 percent did not know how HIV was transmitted, and 73 percent had never use a condom with their regular boyfriends. Nearly 100 percent of students in public secondary schools in Venado Tuerto were sexually active, yet only 20 percent reported regular condom use (Pedrola and others 2000).

A 2000 estimate put the percentage of STI clinic patients infected with HIV at 4.2. Rates among blood donors were lower than the national average, at 0.13 percent (Argentina 2000).

TB is a serious problem in Argentina, which saw high rates among HIV-infected prisoners from 1985 to 1991 (Di Lonardo and others 1995). At a hospital in Buenos Aires, 10 percent of HIV-positive patients had TB between 1987 and 1999 (Nasiff and others 2000). Over half of these were IDUs. Only 7 percent had received preventive treatment with isoniazide, although the mean time between diagnosis of their HIV infection and hospitalization with TB was 30 months. Survival in this group increased after the introduction of highly active antiretroviral therapy (HAART).

Paraguay

Few sources provide information about the HIV/AIDS epidemic in Paraguay. Prenatal testing of pregnant women in 1992 in Asunción identified no HIV-positive pregnant women (UNAIDS 2000s). As of 2001, the prevalence in pregnant women was below 1 percent. Studies of CSWs in Asunción between 1987 and 1990 found 0.1 percent infected with HIV (UNAIDS 2000s), and 0.17 percent of blood donors were reported to be infected in the survey reported in this volume. This survey also indicated that 1 percent of voluntarily tested military recruits and 15 percent of voluntarily tested IDUs were HIV positive. These numbers suggest that the epidemic is more serious than has been acknowledged and that it is concentrated in IDUs rather than in the general heterosexual population and MSM, as official statistics indicate.

Paradoxically, while only 15 percent of 15- to 49-year-olds correctly stated two or more ways to prevent HIV infection, nearly 80 percent of females in this age group were reported to have used a condom during their most recent risky intercourse (UNAIDS 2000s).

Uruguay

Injecting drug use is increasingly significant in the Uruguayan
HIV/AIDS epidemic. Forty percent of babies born with HIV were
born to mothers who injected drugs (*HIV and AIDS in the Americas*
2001; UNAIDS 2000w). Between 1994 and 1997, 15–24 percent of
IDUs in Montevideo tested positive for HIV (UNAIDS 2000y).
Similar rates have been reported in transvestite and male CSWs in
Montevideo in 2000 (*HIV and AIDS in the Americas* 2001); 3.3 percent of the 200 transvestite CSWs surveyed admitted to injecting
drug use, and irregular or no condom use was reported with 22 percent of clients (Serra and others 2000). The government reported that
2 percent of female CSWs and 9 percent of male CSWs aged 15–34
were HIV positive.

Two studies of 12,000 laborers in 1997 and 2000 found 0.23 percent and 0.26 percent, respectively, infected, and among pregnant
women in 2000, 0.23 percent were HIV positive (*HIV and AIDS in
the Americas* 2001). Among blood donors, the rate reported for our
survey was more than twice as high, at 0.6 percent. Luckily, 100 percent of blood donated in Uruguay is screened for HIV (survey data).
In 1993, 6 percent of military recruits were reportedly infected
(survey data), and 6 percent of TB patients in Uruguay had AIDS
(*HIV and AIDS in the Americas* 2001). Regarding the prison population, a local NGO reported that prisoners with AIDS were subjected
to numerous human rights violations, including the suspension of
access to antiretroviral therapy upon incarceration (Viana, Gerschuni,
and Dos Santos 2000).

Chile

Unlike other countries of the Southern Cone, injecting drug use does
not appear to play a large role in HIV transmission in Chile.
Heterosexual transmission is increasing in both men and women and
is especially associated with poverty in women (Chile 2000). The male-
to-female ratio of AIDS cases as of 1997 was 8.4:1, but this ratio is
expected to decrease as the prevalence of cases among MSM decreases.

The highest numbers of AIDS cases by far have been reported in Santiago, followed distantly by Valparaíso and Viña del Mar. Sero-prevalence in gay-identified males in Santiago is estimated to be between 20 percent and 25 percent (Frasca and others 2000). Data on HIV prevalence in IDUs and CSWs are lacking. STI clinic patients tested in 1999 had rates up to 3 percent, with the highest rates in Santiago. HIV prevalence in both pregnant women and blood donors is less than 0.1 percent (UNAIDS 2000e).

Knowledge about HIV prevention is reported to be close to universal among urban 15- to 49-year-olds, and according to one source, condom use during high-risk sex is around 33 percent in this group (UNAIDS 2000e). UNAIDS, WHO, and PAHO reported that, for men, approximately 38 percent of 15- to 19-year-olds, 43 percent of 20- to 29-year-olds, 35 percent of 30- to 39-year-olds, and 33 percent of 40- to 49-year-olds used condoms with casual partners (*HIV and AIDS in the Americas* 2001).

The Economic Impact of HIV/AIDS in Latin America

The economic impact of HIV/AIDS in Latin America manifests itself in several ways, including

- direct costs to government health care systems
- opportunity costs of activities not undertaken by government health care systems
- direct health care costs to PLWHA
- wages lost by PLWHA
- wages lost by caregivers
- indirect costs to society.

Direct costs to government health care systems include the costs of treating PLWHA. These costs can be high on a per-case basis because of the intensity of treatment required for some opportunistic infections and other ailments associated with HIV/AIDS, as well as the relatively high cost of antiretroviral agents prescribed to HIV patients. However, because HIV/AIDS prevalence is not very high in most countries, the overall HIV/AIDS-related resource demands on the public budget have been relatively low to date (only about 0.5–2.6 percent of total health spending in several countries studied).

There are *opportunity costs of activities not undertaken by government health care systems* in favor of spending on HIV/AIDS. The additional resource demands associated with HIV and other emerging health problems in general have not induced more overall health care spending, but rather have led to increased competition among priorities within the health sector. A full economic assessment requires consideration of unmet needs related to spending on HIV/AIDS.

Direct health care costs to PLWHA include out-of-pocket spending on private (and sometimes public) health services and costs paid by insurers.

Wages are lost by PLWHA, who face reduced labor market opportunities because they are unable to work or due to discrimination. Tax revenues are also lost as a result of reduced productivity. Given that HIV/AIDS typically affects people in their most economically active years, lost wages are likely to constitute a large share of the total economic impact of the disease.

Wages lost by caregivers (often family members) of PLWHA are due to additional demands on their time, which detracts from employment.

Indirect costs to society include higher insurance premiums in large populations and lost national income from tourism in areas where high HIV/AIDS prevalence makes locales less desirable to visitors.

Few efforts have been made to estimate the full economic impact of HIV/AIDS in Latin America; this remains on the future policy research agenda.[3] However, several extensive analyses have examined the direct impact of HIV/AIDS on health systems. Preliminary estimates of financing and expenditures in eight Latin American countries in 2000 indicate that the expenditure in Argentina, Bolivia, Brazil, Chile, Costa Rica, Mexico, Peru, and Uruguay on HIV/AIDS was

US$1.13 billion, ranging from US$408,000 in Bolivia to US$579 million in Brazil (Fundación Mexicana de la Salud, SIDALAC, ONUSIDA, and Comisión Europea 2002). The estimated average per capita expenditure devoted to care in Bolivia was 18 percent, but in the other countries it was higher than 64 percent (the average was 78 percent). None of the countries except Bolivia depended heavily on external international cooperation; 25 percent of Bolivia's health expenditure was out-of-pocket expenditures, 64 percent was from external sources, and only a small fraction was covered by direct government funding.

In the seven countries where the government provides antiretroviral therapy, most financing is provided by government resources through universal health systems (e.g., Brazil) or social security institutions.

Latin America spends large proportions on treatment—between 60 percent and 80 percent of total HIV/AIDS expenditures. The majority of countries, such as Brazil, Argentina, Chile, Uruguay, and Mexico, allocate substantial resources to antiretroviral drugs while spending only 10 percent to 30 percent of the total expenditure on prevention (table 1.4).

The vast majority of HIV/AIDS expenditures are financed by public sources. This includes direct government (i.e., ministries of health) or social security contributions, as in Argentina, Brazil, and Costa Rica. In Mexico, Chile, Peru, and Uruguay, the private sector contributes more to HIV/AIDS expenditures, primarily through out-of-pocket-expenditures (table 1.5).

Regarding prevention, the fact that a large portion of expenditures on condoms are financed out of pocket (e.g., Uruguay) means that prevention interventions led by governments might be successful since it is proved that people are willing to invest in priority prevention methods. Conversely, this high level of out-of-pocket expenditures for personal health care services demonstrates the lack of governments' ability or willingness to finance services for people suffering a potentially devastating disease from the economic perspective, not to mention a lack of attention to one of the major causes of morbidity and premature mortality.

Table 1.4. Basic Indicators of Context and Expenditure in Selected Countries, 1999

CONTEXT INDICATOR	ARGENTINA	BOLIVIA	BRAZIL	CHILE	COSTA RICA	MEXICO	PERU	URUGUAY
GDP US$ billion	283.2	8.3	751.5	67.5	15.1	483.7	51.9	20.8
GDP US$ billion (PPP)	449.1	19.2	1,182.0	129.9	31.8	801.3	116.6	29.4
GDP per capita US$ (PPP)	12,277	2,355	7,037	8,652	8,860	8,297	4,622	8,879
Population (millions)	36.6	8.1	168.2	15	3.9	97.4	25.2	3.3
Total expenditure on HIV/AIDS (US$ million)	219,885	408	579,331	52,407	10,190	207,217	42,869	19,825
Structure indicators and expenditure weight (%)								
National health expenditure/GDP (%)	9.1	4.65	7.6	5.8	6.7	5.6	3.1	10.70
Public health expenditure/national health expenditure (%)	21.7	81.3	42.1	46.6	77.6	45.0	40.0	46.3
Total expenditure on AIDS/national health expenditure (%)	0.8	0.92	1.4	1.27	—	0.5	2.6	0.87
Public expenditure on AIDS/health public expenditure (%)	2.2	0.02	2.5	0.7	—	0.96	1.5	0.64
Public expenditure on AIDS/total AIDS expenditure (%)	57.5	2.09	79.3	28.4	67.7	86.01	22.2	34.03
Family expenditure on AIDS/total AIDS expenditure (%)	—	22.64	15.0	66.9	0.6	11.52	74.9	45.13
Condom expenditure per capita (US$ PPP)	1.91	0.03	0.05	0.08	1.23	0.13	0.16	2.69
Antiretrovirals expenditure (US$ PPP)	4.12	0.0	2.73	4.93	2.36	2.22	0.13	3.32
Expenditure composition (%)								
Personnel health	77.9	18.0	72.0	88.5	67.6	83.0	91.9	64.4
Public health and prevention	22.1	53.3	28.0	11.5	32.4	17.0	8.1	35.6

— Not available.

Note: GDP = gross domestic product; PPP = (adjustments made for) parity of purchasing power.

Source: Fundación Mexicana de la Salud, SIDALAC, ONUSIDA, and Comisión Europea 2002.

Table 1.5. AIDS Care Financing by Source in Selected Countries (US$, adjusted for PPP)

FINANCING SOURCE	ARGENTINA	BOLIVIA	BRAZIL	CHILE	COSTA RICA	MEXICO	PERU	URUGUAY
Public sources	200,524	8	706,205	28,655	14,520	22,347	20,088	9,442
Government funds	200,524	8	706,205	15,857	211	35,755	10,193	9,268
Social security funds	n.a.	n.a.	n.a.	12,798	14,309	186,612	9,895	174
Private sources	148,121	282	197,523	71,993	6,941	28,928	74,960	18,580
Private social security	58,368	n.a.	n.a.	n.a.	n.a.	n.a.	n.a.	5,633
Private insurance	19,328	0	—	5,962	n.a.	0	n.a.	n.a.

— Not available.

Note: n.a. = not applicable; PPP = (adjustments made for) parity of purchasing power.
Source: Fundación Mexicana de la Salud, SIDALAC, ONUSIDA, and Comisión Europea 2002.

Notes

1. Caribbean countries are not included in this study, but in many Caribbean countries the epidemic is generalized.

2. In 1985, Mexico passed a law ensuring the safety of blood, after which the incidence of cases due to contaminated blood decreased dramatically.

3. Studies have examined the macroeconomic impact of AIDS in Africa. However, the epidemiological, demographic, and socioeconomic differences between Africa and Latin America preclude any extrapolation from these findings.

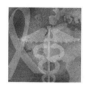

CHAPTER 2

Epidemiological Surveillance

Summary

This chapter assesses the performance of epidemiological surveillance systems as assessed by our survey of informants from 17 Latin American countries. Information on procedures and methodology was provided by technicians in charge of epidemiological surveillance at the national level. In Latin America, cases of HIV and AIDS are reported extensively, although case definition varies among and even within countries. Generally, physicians are responsible for reporting HIV/AIDS cases to health authorities, although in some countries other professionals or entities are involved.

The most common form of case identification is name based, followed by various types of codes. Respondents from each country confirmed that they have laws protecting access to such information, but the existing legislation shows a lack of laws or regulation regarding ownership of surveillance data, information security, and citizens' rights.

Both underreporting and delays in notification compromise the quality and validity of information available. The epidemic in Latin America probably includes about 30 percent more cases of AIDS and 40 percent more cases of HIV than are currently estimated. Generally, active surveillance is not being implemented in most countries.

Sentinel surveillance is an indispensable tool for designing, implementing, and evaluating prevention interventions targeted to all populations. Despite the fact that sentinel surveillance systems are widespread in Latin America, consistent and comparable data are not generated regionwide. Policies for promoting free and anonymous HIV testing and ensuring availability and access to testing are basic conditions for expanding and improving prevention strategies and surveillance plans.

Regarding the information systems currently in place, there is a need to improve the systems for reporting cases, particularly in terms of validity and comprehensiveness. Underreporting is one of the most common problems in Latin America. Most of the sentinel surveillance problems are related to the need for systematizing information systems and incorporating new subpopulations. Second-generation surveillance is a challenge to those responsible for surveillance systems, given the current lack of implementation and development. Second-generation surveillance is the monitoring of HIV and high-risk behavior trends over time to inform the development of interventions and evaluation of their impact. It helps researchers better understand the behaviors driving the epidemic in a country, especially among populations at higher risk of infection. Increased resources, technically trained personnel, and political, policy-related support are the primary objectives for improving HIV/AIDS surveillance in Latin America.

Introduction

In Latin America, epidemiological surveillance of HIV/AIDS at the national level began at the same time as the appearance of the first AIDS cases—in the first half of the 1980s. As in the rest of the world, the first surveillance systems recorded cases of AIDS and were later expanded to include HIV. To various degrees, sentinel surveillance of high-risk behavior was incorporated during the 1990s.

Epidemiological surveillance of HIV/AIDS is crucial to the control of the epidemic. Through surveillance, it is possible to measure the frequency and distribution of HIV/AIDS within and among populations, analyze its evolution, and evaluate the effectiveness of prevention efforts. HIV/AIDS surveillance systems are imperative since HIV/AIDS is an infectious disease with serious public health implications; it is distributed heterogeneously throughout populations, but it is also preventable and linked to behavior patterns. As in other regions of the world, the HIV/AIDS epidemic in Latin America has a different history, profile, and pattern within and among various countries (*HIV and AIDS in the Americas* 2001). Therefore, high-quality information and an understanding of the trends and populations most affected are needed for the preparation and focus of prevention and treatment activities.

This chapter assesses HIV/AIDS epidemiological surveillance systems in Latin America, including their capacity to collect, analyze, interpret, and disseminate the information necessary to control the epidemic. Information was obtained through self-administered, semistructured questionnaires aimed at identifying the resources, characteristics, and activities of national surveillance systems, as well as HIV/AIDS-specific surveillance. The questionnaires were given to the persons managing national HIV/AIDS surveillance system, the national AIDS program, or the department of epidemiology in 17 Latin American countries. The response rate was 100 percent, but the level of completion of the questionnaires was variable, making it impossible to carry out a homogenous analysis of Latin America or establish parameters for country-to-region or country-to-country comparisons. However, wherever possible, this chapter presents some potential subregional (Central America, Andean Region, Southern Cone) areas of joint analysis. The collected information is presented in sections addressing resources, activities, policies, and perception of needs.

Resources for HIV/AIDS Surveillance

Allocation of resources and personnel for surveillance has steadily increased since the 1980s. According to the respondents to our survey, in 2000 the average number of full-time HIV/AIDS surveillance

Table 2.1. HIV/AIDS Surveillance Personnel in Latin America, 2000

COUNTRY OR SUBREGION	NUMBER OF FULL-TIME HIV/AIDS SURVEILLANCE PERSONNEL	SURVEILLANCE PERSONNEL WITH HIV/AIDS TRAINING (%)
Mexico	5	100
Central America	2	83
Guatemala	0	0
El Salvador	0	0
Honduras	—	—
Nicaragua	20[a]	—
Costa Rica	2	—
Panama	0	0
Brazil	15	—
Andean Region	9	20
Venezuela, R.B. de	—	—
Colombia	1	—
Ecuador	3	—
Peru	2	—
Bolivia	3	—
Southern Cone	4	75
Argentina	1	—
Paraguay	0	0
Uruguay	2	—
Chile	1	—
Latin America	35	63

— Not available.
a. The data supplied by Nicaragua were not used in calculating the overall values.
Source: Original survey data.

personnel per country was 2.5 in each country except Paraguay, Panama, Guatemala, and El Salvador (see table 2.1). Overall, one out of every four countries had full-time HIV/AIDS surveillance personnel. With the exception of Guatemala, Paraguay, Colombia, Ecuador, Peru, and Bolivia, all countries required surveillance professionals to receive specific training in HIV/AIDS surveillance.

In Latin America, cases of HIV and AIDS are reported extensively. In every country, it is mandatory to report AIDS cases, and in 94 percent of countries HIV cases must also be reported.

Case Definition

The definition of an AIDS case varies throughout the region, both among and within countries. The most frequently used definitions (in 47 percent of countries) are the 1993 definition from the Centers for Disease Control and Prevention (CDC 1992), the European version of this definition (European Centre for the Epidemiological Monitoring of AIDS 1993), or a combination of both (e.g., CDC 1987b; the "Caracas" definition, in Pan American Health Organization [PAHO] 1990). About 33 percent of countries use highly sensitive definitions based on complex clinical criteria (e.g., Caracas; World Health Organization [WHO] 1986; see table 2.2).

Table 2.2. Definitions of AIDS Used in Latin American Reporting, 2000

COUNTRY OR SUBREGION	CDC93[a] (INCLUDES EUROPEAN VERSION[b])	CDC93 + CDC87[c] + CARACAS[d]	CARACAS	OTHER
Mexico	0	0	0	1
Central America	1	2	1	1
Guatemala	—	—	—	—
El Salvador		✓		
Honduras				WHO[e]
Nicaragua			✓	
Costa Rica	✓			
Panama		✓		
Brazil				CDC87 + Caracas + CDC87 modified
Andean Region	1	1	4	0
Venezuela			✓	
Colombia	✓		✓	
Ecuador		✓		
Peru			✓	
Bolivia			✓	
Southern Cone	1	1	0	1
Argentina				CDC87 + WHO
Paraguay	—	—	—	—
Uruguay	✓			
Chile		✓		
Latin America	3	4	5	4

— Not available.

a. *CDC93* refers to the Centers for Disease Control and Prevention (CDC 1992) definition of AIDS.

b. *European version* refers to the European Center for the Epidemiological Monitoring of AIDS (1993) definition of AIDS.

c. *CDC87* refers to the CDC 1987b definition of AIDS.

d. *Caracas* refers to the PAHO (1990) definition of AIDS.

e. *WHO* refers to the WHO (1986) definition of AIDS.

Source: Original survey data.

Use of the 1993 CDC definition requires a developed health infrastructure and sophisticated methods for suitable and appropriate diagnosis (CDC 1992). Possibly for this reason, many countries use this definition in combination with others found to be more adaptable and appropriate for local health resources. The coexistence of different case definitions can generate problems in terms of sensitivity (proportion of cases diagnosed and captured in the system) and predictive value (proportion of cases reported that actually meet the criteria to be counted as a case) (German 2000). HIV case definitions are often based on serologic detection of HIV antibodies, yet the definitions used in many cases are imprecise, nonspecific, and barely conclusive from a clinical point of view (see table 2.3).

Case Reporting

According to our survey data, physicians are most often responsible for reporting HIV/AIDS cases to health authorities, although in some countries other professionals or entities are involved. For example, nongovernmental organizations (NGOs) in El Salvador also report cases, and in Honduras, nurses, social workers, and psychologists also report cases. In Bolivia, diagnostic labs report HIV/AIDS cases, which limits the clinical and sociodemographic information documented about patients. In Panama, the responsibility for notification is delegated to individuals such as physicians, managers of commercial sex workers (CSWs), personnel responsible for medical patients, laboratory workers, or any citizen with knowledge or "suspicion" of HIV/AIDS infection or illness. In every country cases are reported to the national ministry of health either directly or through regional or state offices (figure 2.1).

Active vs. Passive Surveillance

Active surveillance implies that surveillance services search for cases in relevant settings, whereas in *passive surveillance* these services receive and process data reported from elsewhere. Active surveillance has the potential for more comprehensive recording of HIV/AIDS cases, yet

Table 2.3. HIV/AIDS Case Definitions by Country, 2000

COUNTRY	DEFINITION OF HIV CASE
Mexico	Infection with HIV or diagnosis of AIDS with the ability to infect others
Guatemala	—
El Salvador	Double positive results with different types of HIV-reactive tests and positive WB
Honduras	Serologically positive test results for HIV and at least one major symptom characteristic of or associated with AIDS
Nicaragua	Reactive ELISA, confirmed with WB, not necessarily with any symptoms of AIDS
Costa Rica	Reactive ELISA and WB
Panama	Positive, confirmed HIV test
Brazil	2 reactive ELISA from different sources and 1 confirming test (WB, IFA)
Venezuela, R.B. de	—
Colombia	2 reactive ELISA and 1 WB or IFA
Ecuador	Adolescents and adults: 2 reactive ELISA confirmed with IFA or WB, or any test detecting HIV antibodies, HIV antigen, or genetic evidence Children <18 months: positive results in 2 tests (HIV culture, PCR antigen 24)
Peru	—
Bolivia	—
Argentina	Centers for Disease Control and Prevention (CDC) 1993 definition
Paraguay	Adults and children over 18 months: positive serologic test (ELISA, confirmed by WB) without signs or symptoms of AIDS Children under 18 months: PCR (currently not in use)
Uruguay	—
Chile	CDC 1987 definition, diagnostic algorithm established in Chile

— Not available.
Note: ELISA = enzyme-linked immunosorbent assay; IFA = immunofluorescence assay; PCR = polimerase chain reaction; WB = Western Blot. For CDC case definition, see http://www.cdc.gov/epo/dphsi/casedef/acquired_immunodeficiency_syndrome_current.htm. For WHO case definition, see http://www.who.int/emc-documents/surveillance/docs/whocdscsrisr992.html/01Aids.htm. For European case definition, see http://ceses.org. For Caracas AIDS case definition, see http://lac-hiv-epinet.org.
Source: Original survey data.

it is very costly since teams of professionals must travel to sites for data collection. In areas of high incidence of HIV/AIDS, active surveillance generates more sensitive surveillance data (Thacker and others 1986). Active surveillance is used in only seven countries (Mexico, El Salvador, Costa Rica, Peru, Brazil, República Bolivariana de Venezuela, and Uruguay), and the level of use varies.

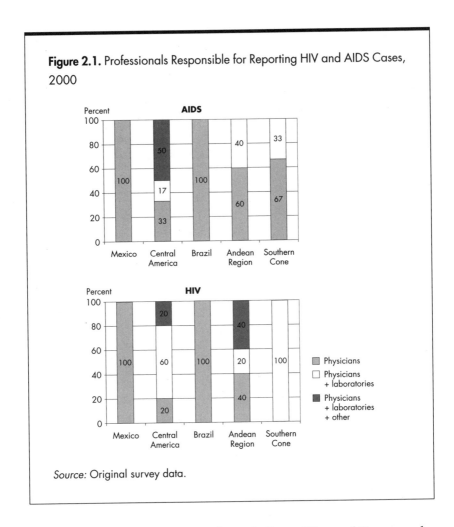

Figure 2.1. Professionals Responsible for Reporting HIV and AIDS Cases, 2000

Source: Original survey data.

According to the data we collected, Costa Rica and Peru are the countries with the most extensive active surveillance of HIV/AIDS cases. The number of countries with active surveillance may actually be fewer than is presented here, since in some instances there was confusion between sentinel surveillance and active surveillance.

Reporting Forms

Standardized case reports help health care professionals keep track of sociodemographic, epidemiological, and clinical information needed

Table 2.4. Countries and Subregions with Reporting Forms for Case Notification, 2000

COUNTRY OR SUBREGION	AIDS CASE REPORTING FORM	HIV CASE REPORTING FORM
Mexico	✓	✓
Central America	6	4
Guatemala	✓	
El Salvador	✓	✓
Honduras	✓	✓
Nicaragua	✓	✓
Costa Rica	✓	
Panama	✓	✓
Brazil	✓	✓
Andean Region	5	1
Venezuela, R.B. de	✓	
Colombia	✓	
Ecuador	✓	
Peru	✓	✓
Bolivia	✓	
Southern Cone	4	1
Argentina	✓	
Paraguay	✓	✓
Uruguay	✓	
Chile	✓	
Latin America	17 (100.0%)	8 (41.1%)

Note: Most countries use the same reporting form to collect data from HIV and AIDS cases.
Source: Original survey data.

to characterize cases. In most countries, there are standardized forms for HIV/AIDS case notification, although standard forms are used more for AIDS case reporting than for HIV reporting (see table 2.4).

Case Identification

The purpose of case identification is to eliminate or reduce duplication of HIV/AIDS cases reported. A common method for identifying cases is through very detailed personal indicators (e.g., name, date of birth, personal identification numbers, or codes), as well as other identifiers that have less discriminatory power (Joint United Nations Programme on HIV/AIDS [UNAIDS] 2000x; Osmond and others 1999; CDC 1999a).

In the majority of countries (9 out of 17) duplication is controlled through case identification by first and last name. In six countries, the most widely used code for identification consists of the person's initials (first and last name) and date of birth. In Colombia, personal identification numbers are used as case identifiers, and initials are most frequently used in the Southern Cone and Central America (table 2.5).

Like all surveillance systems, those designed for HIV/AIDS require a case identification mechanism to prevent reporting duplication; however, the question of patient confidentiality may be raised. Information systems containing personal data (names, codes, or others) may ultimately be sensitive enough to identify specific people, yet to carry out public health and assistance activities, health

Table 2.5. Case Identifiers Used in HIV/AIDS Reporting, 2000

COUNTRY OR SUBREGION	IDENTIFIERS USED
Mexico	Name
Central America	Name (50%), Code (50%)
Guatemala	Code
El Salvador	Name
Honduras	Name
Nicaragua	Code
Costa Rica	Code
Panama	Name
Brazil	Name
Andean Region	Name (60%), Code (40%)
Venezuela, R. B. de	Name
Colombia	Personal identification number
Ecuador	Name
Peru	Code
Bolivia	Name
Southern Cone	Name (25%), Code (75%)
Argentina	Code
Paraguay	Code
Uruguay	Name
Chile	Code
Latin America	Name (53%), Code (47%)

Source: Original survey data.

administrators often require access to this personal information. This issue clearly points to the need for secure, well-protected information systems that guarantee patients' rights to confidentiality and privacy.

Each country's respondents confirmed that there are laws protecting access to such information. In some countries, these laws directly relate to HIV/AIDS cases, while in others they are incorporated in rules for public health activities and standards for professional conduct. In a few countries these laws loosely exist in the Constitution or legislation but are not specifically health related (see table 2.6). In reviewing the existing legislation, it is interesting to note the scarcity of laws regarding ownership of surveillance data, information security, and citizens' rights.

Table 2.6. Legislation Regarding Confidentiality Issues

COUNTRY	CONFIDENTIALITY LEGISLATION
Mexico	NOM 10 and NOM 17
Guatemala	
El Salvador	Professional ethics law
Honduras	Special law for HIV/AIDS, articles 58, 60 and 61
Nicaragua	Nonspecific legislation
Costa Rica	General AIDS law
Panama	Law 3 of 5 January 2000
Brazil	Law for information protection, nonspecific
Venezuela, R.B. de	Resolution for respecting rights to confidentiality
Colombia	Decree 1543 of June 1997
Ecuador	Statistics law
Peru	Information protection law: Anti-AIDS Law 26626
Bolivia	No law for information protection
Argentina	Law 23.798/90–Article 2(a)
Paraguay	Law #102/91 (in revision)
Uruguay	No specific law; rights recognized in the constitution Personal information protected by the law of the ministry of public health
Chile	Decree for obligatory reporting of infectious diseases (#712, article 4 of November 1999) Law for information protection, nonspecific

Note: Information in this table reflects answers given on the questionnaire.
NOM = *Normas Oficiales Mexicanas.*
Source: Original survey data.

Underreporting and Delays in Notification

Both underreporting (i.e., cases diagnosed but not reported to the national or local registries) and delays in notification compromise the quality and validity of information available. It is possible to make mathematical predictions to compensate for delays in notification, yet underreporting is still a serious limiting factor that results in under-estimation of the true magnitude of the HIV/AIDS epidemic.

The time period between diagnosis of a case and reporting to national or local registries varies. According to respondents, in most countries, the turnaround time is about three to six months, except in Chile and Panama, where over six months is the norm, and Mexico and Colombia, where the longest delays were found of over a year between diagnosis and appearance of the case in the surveillance system (table 2.7).

Underreporting in Latin America is high, with an average of 54.8 percent of HIV cases and 43.5 percent of AIDS cases not reported, according to results from this survey. The lowest levels of underre-porting were found in Brazil, Uruguay, Chile, and Argentina, and the highest levels were in Colombia, Guatemala, and Honduras. Region-ally, Central America and the Andean Region have the highest levels of underreporting. Not every country estimates the number of cases underreported (i.e., Ecuador, Peru, República Bolivariana de Venezuela, and Paraguay), and HIV underreporting receives less attention than underreporting of AIDS. Based on the data collected for this study, the epidemic in Latin America probably includes about 30 percent more cases of AIDS and 40 percent more cases of HIV than are currently estimated.

All countries in Latin America distribute periodic bulletins about the distribution and evolution of the HIV/AIDS epidemic. Infor-mation about AIDS is more systematized than information about HIV. Bulletins are usually disseminated quarterly or biannually, although Colombia issues more frequent bulletins on the spread of HIV/AIDS and Brazil does the same for HIV. Most countries dis-tribute information about both HIV and AIDS, but some provide information only on AIDS (Guatemala, Paraguay, and Panama), and

Table 2.7. Underreporting and Delays in Notification, 2000

COUNTRY OR SUBREGION	DELAY IN HIV REPORTING				DELAY IN AIDS REPORTING			HIV UNDERREPORTING	AIDS UNDERREPORTING
	<6 MO.	6 MONTHS–1 YEAR	>1 YEAR	—	<6 MONTHS	6 MONTHS–1 YEAR	>1 YEAR		
Mexico			✓				✓	91.2%[a]	18.5%[a]
Central America	50.0%	17.0%	0.0%	33.0%	83.0%	17.0%	0.0%	43.3%	33.2%
Guatemala	✓				✓			—	50.0%
El Salvador	✓				✓			40.0%	40.0%
Honduras	✓				✓			—	47.0%
Nicaragua				✓	✓			60.0%	30.0%
Costa Rica		✓						30.0%	30.0%
Panama						✓		—	32.0%
Brazil	✓				✓			—	7.0%
Andean Region	80.0%		20.0%		80.0%		20.0%	70.0%	55.0%
Venezuela, R.B. de	✓		✓		✓			—	—
Colombia							✓	80.0%	80.0%
Ecuador	✓				✓			—	—
Peru	✓				✓			—	—
Bolivia	✓				✓			60.0%	30.0%
Southern Cone	50.0%			50.0%	75.0%	25.0%		15.0%	14.0%
Argentina				✓	✓			—	20.0%
Paraguay	✓				✓			—	—
Uruguay	✓			✓		✓		15.0%	10.0%
Chile								—	14.0%
Latin America	59.0%	6.0%	12.0%	23.0%	76.0%	12.0%	12.0%	54.8%	43.6%

— Not available.

a. Last estimates from Mexico 2002.

Source: Original survey data.

in Costa Rica, based on the questionnaire response, it seems that this epidemiological information is not disseminated at all.

In most countries, HIV/AIDS data are distributed to the appropriate health administrations, health care professionals, universities, NGOs, researchers, and the general media (table 2.8). Only the respondents from Paraguay and El Salvador said that information

Table 2.8. Professionals and Organizations Receiving Epidemiological Information on HIV/AIDS, 2000

PROFESSIONAL OR ORGANIZATION	RECEIVE AIDS INFORMATION ONLY	RECEIVE HIV/AIDS INFORMATION	RECEIVE NO INFORMATION
Administrators	Guatemala, Panama, Venezuela, R.B. de	Mexico, El Salvador, Honduras, Nicaragua, Colombia, Ecuador, Peru, Brazil, Argentina, Uruguay, Chile	
Physicians	Guatemala, Panama, Venezuela, R.B. de	Mexico, El Salvador, Honduras, Brazil, Colombia, Ecuador, Peru, Argentina, Uruguay, Chile	Paraguay
Nurses	Guatemala, Panama	Mexico, El Salvador, Honduras, Brazil, Colombia, Chile	Paraguay
Universities	Guatemala, Panama	Honduras, Nicaragua, Brazil, Colombia, Peru, Argentina, Chile	El Salvador, Paraguay
Nongovernmental organizations	Guatemala, Panama, Venezuela, R.B. de	Mexico, El Salvador, Honduras, Nicaragua, Brazil, Colombia, Ecuador, Peru, Argentina, Uruguay, Chile	
Researchers	Guatemala, Panama	Mexico, Honduras, Nicaragua, Brazil, Colombia, Ecuador, Bolivia, Argentina, Chile	El Salvador, Paraguay
Press and media	Guatemala, Panama, Venezuela, R.B. de, Paraguay	Mexico, El Salvador, Honduras, Nicaragua, Brazil, Colombia, Bolivia, Ecuador, Argentina, Uruguay, Chile	

Source: Original survey data.

regarding HIV/AIDS is not provided to professionals or researchers. In general, the survey respondents felt that wide distribution is useful since health care workers are better informed about the profile of the epidemic, there is greater collaboration among health care authorities, and more interventions are planned as a result of the information contained in the bulletins and reports. The majority of countries maintain HIV- and AIDS-related data at the national level (ministries of health), while less information on HIV and AIDS is available at the local or regional level. This gap is especially notable in the Southern Cone (see table 2.9). Most respondents felt that distribution of HIV/AIDS epidemiological information to the national government was very valuable for decision making, most notably regarding the

Table 2.9. Systematization of HIV and AIDS Records, 2000

COUNTRY OR SUBREGION	SYSTEMATIZATION OF HIV DATA		SYSTEMATIZATION OF AIDS DATA	
	NATIONAL MINISTRY OF HEALTH	LOCAL	NATIONAL MINISTRY OF HEALTH	LOCAL
Mexico	✓	✓	✓	✓
Central America	5 (83%)	4 (67%)	6 (100%)	4 (67%)
Guatemala	—		✓	
El Salvador	✓	✓	✓	✓
Honduras	✓	✓	✓	✓
Nicaragua	✓		✓	
Costa Rica	✓	✓	✓	✓
Panama	✓	✓	✓	✓
Brazil	✓	✓	✓	✓
Andean Region	5 (100%)	3 (60%)	5 (100%)	3 (60%)
Venezuela	✓	✓	✓	✓
Colombia	✓	✓	✓	✓
Ecuador	✓		✓	
Peru	✓		✓	
Bolivia	✓	✓	✓	✓
Southern Cone	4 (100%)	1 (25%)	4 (100%)	1 (25%)
Argentina	✓	✓	✓	✓
Paraguay	✓		✓	
Uruguay	✓		✓	
Chile	✓		✓	
Latin America	16 (94%)	10 (59%)	17 (100%)	10 (59%)

— Not available.
Source: Original survey data.

design, implementation, and expansion of prevention programs, and in increasing the resources allocated to fighting the epidemic.

Surveillance Activities

Evaluation of Surveillance Systems

According to those surveyed, 65 percent of the countries had carried out evaluations of their epidemiological surveillance systems and registries of AIDS and HIV cases. In some countries these evaluations were carried out periodically (Honduras, Nicaragua, Mexico, Peru, Bolivia, and Brazil), while in other countries these evaluations had not been carried out at all (El Salvador, Costa Rica, Panama, República Bolivariana de Venezuela, Colombia, and Paraguay). In the process of administering the surveys and collecting data, there appears to have been some confusion between actual evaluations of the surveillance systems and reports on the balance and trends of the HIV epidemic. The respondents indicated that the results of the evaluations carried out systematically in some countries were not always well supported, and in some cases the evaluations did not correspond to true evaluation studies, but rather to reports on the status and evolution of the epidemic in the country.

Sentinel Surveillance

Sentinel surveillance systems for HIV/AIDS provide more detailed information on the scope of the epidemic and its evolution in various subpopulations. For this reason, sentinel surveillance is an indispensable tool in the design, implementation, and evaluation of prevention interventions targeted to high-risk or variable risk populations (Pappaioanou and others 1990; Onorato, Jones, and Forrester 1990; WHO and UNAIDS 2000). Most of the countries surveyed (14 out of 17) had structured systems for sentinel surveillance of HIV/AIDS integrated into the overall HIV/AIDS information system; the República Bolivariana de Venezuela, Costa Rica, and Panama were the exceptions. The populations prioritized and targeted by sentinel surveillance (by order of frequency) were CSWs, pregnant women, men who have sex with men (MSM), and patients with sexually transmitted infections (STIs). Although structured systems exist in most countries, only the respondents from Argentina, Ecuador, Mexico, Brazil, and Uruguay had information on the priority, high-risk populations. The most logical explanation for this gap is that many of the other countries only recently implemented sentinel surveillance, so information should be expected in the near future. In most countries, HIV/AIDS prevalence was estimated by collecting the results of voluntary tests in various testing and diagnosis centers. Unlinked anonymous testing is commonly used for blood collected for diagnostic purposes.

Our survey found that despite the fact that sentinel surveillance systems are widespread in Latin America, consistent data are lacking. However, most of the estimates of HIV/AIDS prevalence are based on results of studies carried out at various points in time, in different areas, and by different institutions. The often disparate estimates generated by sentinel surveillance of HIV prevalence are shown in detail in table 2.10.

High-quality information on HIV/AIDS prevalence in Latin America is hard to come by and misleading or contradictory. This survey found that there are wide differences among estimates available for the countries, which could be an effect of the various methods or procedures used by the country and international organizations (UNAIDS, PAHO, and WHO) to produce them (UNAIDS 2000w; PAHO 2000c).

Overall, it can be said that there is a high prevalence of HIV in most high-risk Latin American populations. The highest rates among CSWs were in Honduras (10 percent of CSWs), while much lower rates were found in Peru (1.6 percent), Argentina (1.9 percent), and Paraguay (less than 2 percent). The prevalence among transvestites in Uruguay (21 percent) is alarming.

There is very little information on STI patients in Latin America. This is a major concern, considering their high prevalence in all countries and the fact that STI infections are a key risk factor for

Table 2.10. Results of HIV Sentinel Surveillance Studies

COUNTRY OR SUBREGION	POPULATION	METHOD	POPULATION SIZE	ESTIMATED PREVALENCE (%)	DATE OF START
Mexico	Hospital population	VT	19,286	0.35	1992
	Prisoners (men)	VT	5,751	1.4	1985
	Prisoners (men)	VT	798	3.1	1991
	Pregnant women	VT	12,068	0.09	1990
	IDUs	VT	1,816	4.13	1987
	CSWs (female)	VT	38,347	0.59	1987
	CSWs (male)	VT	15,784	4.41	1987
	Blood donors	OT	992,586	0.007	1986
Guatemala	—	—	—	—	—
El Salvador	—	—	—	—	—
Honduras	Pregnant women	ANL/VT	3.248	1.4	1998
	Prisoners	ANL/VT	2.095	6.8	1997
	CSWs	ANL/VT	699	9.9	1998
	Night watchmen	ANL/VT	200	0.5	1998
	Garífuna population	ANL/VT	310	8.4	1998
	MSM	ANL/VT	422	8	1998
	Truck drivers	ANL/VT	458	1.1	1998
Nicaragua	CSWs	ANL	400	0.02	1998
	Blood donors	VT	1500	0.07	—
	TB patients	ANL	760	0.52	—
	STI patients	ANL	—	—	1999
	Pregnant women	VT	—	—	2001
	CSWs	ANL	—	—	2001
	Blood donors	VT	—	—	—
Costa Rica	—	—	—	—	—
Panama	Pregnant women	ANL			
	Newborns' mothers	ANL			
	Prisoners	VT	879	5.8	1991
	Blood donors	OT	—	—	—
	CSWs	OT	—	—	—
Brazil	STI patients	ANL	2,748	4.7	1999
	Pregnant women	ANL	15,226	0.6	2000
	Prisoners	ANL	—	—	—
	CSWs	ANL	—	—	—
	Blood donors	OT	—	—	—
Venezuela, R.B. de	Pregnant women	VT	—	—	1999
	Blood donors				
Colombia	MSM	—	—	18	1999
	STI patients	ANL	4375	<2	1999
	Pregnant women	ANL	8690	<1	1999
	General medicine patients	ANL	9004	<1	1999

(table continued on next page)

Table 2.10. (continued)

COUNTRY OR SUBREGION	POPULATION	METHOD	POPULATION SIZE	ESTIMATED PREVALENCE (%)	DATE OF START
Ecuador	CSWs	VT	100 per year	—	1999
	MSM	VT	100 per year	—	1999
	Pregnant women	VT	5000	0.05	2001
Peru	STI patients	ANL	—	7	1997
	Pregnant women	ANL	—	0.3	2000
	Blood donors	OT	—	0.01	2000
	CSWs	ANL	—	1.6	1999
	Prisoners	*ANL*	—	—	—
	Pregnant women	*ANL*	—	—	—
Bolivia	Hospital population	ANL	784	0.02	2000
	STI patients	ANL	784	0.03	2000
	Pregnant women	ANL	784	—	2000
	CSWs	ANL	784	0.03	2000
Argentina	*STI patients*	*VT*	*320*	*4.16*	*2000*
	Pregnant women	*VT*	*96,011*	*0.66*	*2000*
	Prisoners	*VT*	*2,017*	*17.55*	*2000*
	IDUs	*VT*	*157*	*45.8*	*2000*
	Army volunteers	*VT*	*27,011*	*3.23*	*2000*
	CSWs			*1.9*	
Paraguay	Pregnant women	ANL		<1	—
	Prisoners	VT	—	1	—
	CSWs	VT	—	<2	—
	Blood donors	OT	—	0.17	—
	IDUs	VT	—	15	—
	Health care workers	VT	—	0	—
Uruguay	Pregnant women	VT	2,000	0.23	2000
	Prisoners	VT		6	1993
	CSWs	VT	500	0.45	1995
	CSWs	VT	300	0.35	2000
	Transvestites	VT	200	21	2000
	Employed population	*ANL*	*12,000*	*0.23*	*1996*
	Pregnant women	*VT*	*2,000 per year*	*0.23*	*1991*
	Blood donors	*OT*	*120,000*	*0.6*	*1988*
Chile	STI patients	ANL	—	—	—
	Pregnant women	ANL	—	—	—
	CSWs	VT	—	—	—
	TB patients	VT	—	—	—
	Pregnant women	*ANL*	—	—	—

— Not available.

Note: Epidemiological surveillance system data are in italics for comparison with other different surveys. ANL = unlinked anonymous testing; CSW = commercial sex worker; IDU = injecting drug user; MSM = men who have sex with men; OT = obligatory testing; STI = sexually transmitted infection; TB = tuberculosis; VT = voluntary testing.

contracting HIV. High prevalence rates were found in Peru (7 percent) and Argentina (4.16 percent), while lower rates were found in Colombia (less than 2 percent) and Bolivia (0.03 percent). There are no data available from Central America, although a multicenter study is currently projected by different organizations and information will be available soon.

Prisoners show high prevalence rates in Central America (Honduras and Panama) and the Southern Cone (Argentina and Uruguay), possibly due to the high numbers of injecting drug users (IDUs) in prison. Although they are considered one of the highest risk groups for transmission, there are very few sentinel studies on IDUs in prisons. Estimates of prevalence within IDU populations in Argentina (46 percent) and Paraguay (15 percent) demonstrate the high-risk nature of injecting drug use and the urgent need for monitoring.

MSM are one of the least studied populations in Latin America, despite the fact that in most countries they represent the majority of AIDS cases and are considered a priority group for HIV sentinel surveillance. Honduras has data available on this population, yet even in this country the data are questionable (the estimate of an 8 percent prevalence rate among MSM in Honduras could be too low). In Colombia, HIV prevalence among MSM is estimated at 18 percent (1999–2000 data).

These high-risk populations act as a reservoir for the epidemic and are key players in the spread of infection, but they have not yet been the focus of systematic, periodic studies (World Bank 1997). Due to the scarcity of data, analysis of the current status of the epidemic and its geographic and over-time trends becomes difficult. Subsequently, development of proper interventions for the country or from a regional perspective becomes a difficult task.

Sentinel studies of groups with variable risk (e.g., truck drivers, hospital populations) and others with about the same risk as the general population (e.g., employees, pregnant women) are surprisingly common in Latin America. In some countries, studies of variable risk populations are more numerous and extensive than those of high-risk populations, in which monitoring infection patterns could have a greater impact on prevention and control. Since variable risk populations have relatively low prevalence rates, the studies designed for them are often larger in scope and more costly.

The highest prevalence rates among variable risk groups are found in Honduras (1.1 percent in truck drivers, 8.4 percent in Garífunas, and 1.4 percent in pregnant women). Prevalence rates among pregnant women range from 0.05 percent in Ecuador to less than 1 percent in Colombia and Paraguay. The prevalence of 3.23 percent among army volunteers in Argentina is notable and is possibly the result of a high level of injecting drug use in this population. In some countries, blood donors have greater prevalence rates than the general population. For instance, in Uruguay, prevalence is 0.23 percent in the employed population and 0.6 percent among blood donors.

According to the survey results, most countries (11 out of 17) have estimates of the number of people living with HIV, although many do not report the sources or publish the methods used. Some countries use UNAIDS, WHO, or PAHO estimates, while others obtain estimates through sentinel studies that are not necessarily representative of the general population or calculations with unclear scientific validity. None of the estimates are derived from the most common methods for estimating prevalence (Hughes, Porter, and Gill 1998; Karon, Khare, and Rosenberg 1998). In turn, estimates of people living with HIV range from 0.22 per 1,000 in the República Bolivariana de Venezuela to 0.02 per 1,000 in Bolivia. According to the data presented, the prevalence in Honduras was 0.38 per 1,000, while in Panama it was 8.2 per 1,000, but these estimates are not coherent with the expected dimensions of the epidemic in each country or with estimates from international organizations (see table 2.11). These estimates and those from sentinel surveillance systems are not comparable with epidemiological data supplied by regional authorities and studies. Therefore, the República Bolivariana de Venezuela would be the most affected country, surpassing Brazil and Honduras.

Behavior Surveillance

According to our survey responses, seven of the 17 countries had conducted knowledge, attitude, and practice (KAP) surveys in recent

Table 2.11. People Living with HIV, December 2000

COUNTRY OR SUBREGION	NUMBER OF PERSONS LIVING WITH HIV[a]	PERSONS LIVING WITH HIV/100,000[b]	NUMBER OF PERSONS LIVING WITH HIV[c]	PERSONS LIVING WITH HIV/100,000[c]
Mexico	116,000	117.29	150,000	151.67
Central America	29,971	307.21	196,900	525.11
Guatemala	—	—	73,000	640.35
El Salvador	3,444	54.66	20,000	317.46
Honduras	2,500	38.46	63,000	969.23
Nicaragua	—	—	4,900	96.08
Costa Rica	—	—	12,000	300.00
Panama	24,027	828.51	24,000	827.59
Brazil	597,000	350.97	540,000	317.46
Andean Region	634,627	631.46	204,200	74.25
Venezuela, R.B. de	540,000	2,231.40	62,000	256.20
Colombia	18,429	44.36	71,000	167.85
Ecuador	—	—	19,000	150.79
Peru	76,000	295.71	48,000	186.77
Bolivia	198	2.38	4,200	50.60
Southern Cone	143,517	208.49	154,000	130.93
Argentina	122,000	329.72	130,000	351.35
Paraguay	—	—	3,000	54.55
Uruguay	6,500	196.96	6,000	181.82
Chile	15,017	98.79	15,000	98.68
Latin America	1,514,825	381.13	1,245,100	301.08

— = Not available.
a. Figures reflect data given by national respondents.
b. Figures were calculated from data given by national respondents.
c. Data are from UNAIDS 2000k.

years. The populations studied most were the general population and young people (in Peru, Brazil, Paraguay, Uruguay, and Chile), while high-risk populations were studied only in Uruguay (transvestites and IDUs), Brazil (CSWs, IDUs, and people of low socioeconomic status), Peru (MSM), and Chile (STI patients). Currently, Mexico is the only country collecting information on adolescent high-risk behaviors through sentinel sites. The most recent high-risk behavior studies took place in Peru (Endes 2000; CER 1999), Brazil (various populations in 2000–01), and Uruguay (transvestites).

Respondents from 11 countries stated that they had surveillance system plans for high-risk HIV-related behaviors; the most common target populations were MSM and female CSWs. In Mexico, Argentina, Brazil, and Colombia, IDUs and male CSWs were also targeted (Nicaragua's system also covers male CSWs). In Honduras, there was no plan for behavior surveillance, although some studies of MSM and female CSWs have been carried out. El Salvador, Panama, and Costa Rica had no information on prevalence of high-risk behaviors or plan for behavior surveillance. Instead, many have plans for future studies or are focusing efforts on ensuring continuity among studies carried out in past years. Among these countries, only three (Brazil, Argentina, and Paraguay) have concrete plans to identify behavior patterns in high-risk groups (i.e., MSM, CSWs, prisoners, and IDUs).

Participation of other institutions or researchers in these studies is rare. Universities are sometimes involved, but often these studies are carried out exclusively by ministries of health.

HIV Testing and Diagnosis Policies

Policies for promoting HIV testing, as well as facilitating availability and access to the test, are basic conditions for any prevention, diagnosis, or surveillance plan. Epidemiologists in 12 of the 17 countries reported that HIV testing was free, yet this information is not consistent with reports from NGOs and physicians in these countries. For instance, in Peru, Colombia, Ecuador, Panama, and Guatemala, the test is supposed to be free, but people must pay for the diagnosis (often carried out in a separate laboratory), according to the same sources.

Availability of Services for HIV Diagnosis

According to the data collected for this survey, with the exception of Bolivia and Guatemala, local laboratories are used to diagnose HIV, although all tests confirmed with Western Blot or immunofluorescence assay or another test are analyzed centrally. Seven countries confirmed positive tests in national laboratories (El Salvador, Honduras,

Table 2.12. Availability of Laboratories and Centers for Anonymous Diagnosis, 2000

COUNTRY OR SUBREGION	NUMBER OF HIV DIAGNOSTIC LABORATORIES/100,000 INHABITANTS	NUMBER OF ANONYMOUS DIAGNOSTIC CENTERS FOR HIV
Mexico	0.31	22
Central America		
Guatemala	—	—
El Salvador	0.49	—
Honduras	0.55	—
Nicaragua	0.49	17
Costa Rica	—	1
Panama	0.01	—
Brazil	0.30	208
Andean Region		
Venezuela, R.B. de	0.11	—
Colombia	—	—
Ecuador	0.47	—
Peru	—	—
Bolivia	0.03	3
Southern Cone		
Argentina	7.51	14
Paraguay	0.40	—
Uruguay	2.0	—
Chile	—	3

— Not available.
Source: Original survey data.

Nicaragua, Peru, Chile, Paraguay, and Mexico). Information on availability and coverage of national laboratories is scarce and occasionally found to be inconsistent. Estimates show variations in the number of laboratories per 100,000 inhabitants from 0.001 in Panama to 7.5 in Argentina, averaging 1.13 per 100,000 inhabitants (table 2.12).

Availability of anonymous diagnosis centers for high-risk populations is crucial for prevention and diagnosis and for HIV counseling (PAHO 1999b). According to the survey findings, eight countries (Brazil, Mexico, Costa Rica, Nicaragua, Guatemala, Argentina, Chile, and Bolivia) had such centers. Surprisingly, Honduras, the country most affected by the epidemic, did not have anonymous HIV diagnosis centers.

Cost of HIV Testing and Diagnosis

It was not possible to estimate an average overall cost for HIV testing from the information obtained from the participants in the study; data available from public and private centers are inconsistent and vary greatly. A significant difference was observed in the costs of testing in the public sector versus the private sector. The cost of HIV testing in Latin America ranged from US$0 to US$7 in public centers and from US$4 to US$22.85 in private centers (table 2.13). The median cost was US$8.00 in public centers and US$12.50 in private centers.

Table 2.13. Cost of HIV Testing in Public and Private Health Centers, 2000

COUNTRY OR SUBREGION	COST OF HIV TEST IN PRIVATE CENTERS (US$)	COST OF HIV TEST IN PUBLIC CENTERS (US$)
Mexico	—	—
Central America		
Guatemala	—	—
El Salvador	22.85	5.71
Honduras	13.00	—
Nicaragua	10.00	—
Costa Rica	—	—
Panama	20.00	7.00
Brazil	—	free
Andean Region		
Venezuela, R.B. de	—	—
Colombia	20.00	0.43
Ecuador	12.00	5.00
Peru	12.00	6.00
Bolivia	4.00	1.00
Southern Cone		
Argentina	15.00	3.00
Paraguay	15.00	—
Uruguay	10.00	—
Chile	6.50	—
Latin America (average)	13.36	4.02

— Not available.
Source: Original survey data.

Frequency of HIV Testing

Data regarding the frequency of HIV testing were few and disparate, ranging from 77 tests per 1,000 inhabitants in Uruguay to 2.32 per 1,000 in Mexico. Frequency of HIV testing has risen since 1996 in almost all countries, and based on the information available, it seems that it continues to rise. For example, the number of HIV tests carried out per 1,000 people in the República Bolivariana de Venezuela doubled from 1996 to 2000, from 4.13 to 8.26, and increased dramatically in Argentina and Chile, from 0.81 and 0.12 to 12.08 and 15.98, respectively. Uruguay is the country with the most frequent HIV testing, with an average of 77 per 1,000 people.

Blood Supply Safety

Policies for preventing HIV transmission through medical procedures requiring blood or blood products are the responsibility of each country's national health system. To this end, universal screening of donated blood as well as voluntary, altruistic donation must be universally accepted norms (PAHO 1999a). According to our survey and published data, 10 out of the 17 countries reported screening 100 percent of the blood supply (there were no data from two countries; see figure 2.2). The Andean Region had the lowest rate of screening of donated blood, primarily due to the very low rates of screening in Bolivia. According to the data collected, coverage of blood screening is comparable between Central America and the Southern Cone (figure 2.2).

HIV prevalence among blood donors in Latin America is very high (0.19 percent), according to this survey, with the highest prevalence found in Uruguay. In some countries, these high rates among blood donors could be related to policies for blood donation that provide compensation or HIV testing. Study findings indicate that in some cases, HIV prevalence rates among blood donors are higher than estimates for the general population. Only Honduras, Argentina, and Brazil had policies allowing only voluntary, altruistic blood donations.

Table 2.14. Policies for Accepting Blood Donations, 2000

VOLUNTARY, ALTRUISTIC	REPLACEMENT DONORS	VOLUNTARY AND ALTRUISTIC PLUS OTHER POLICY
Honduras	Bolivia	Mexico
Brazil	Chile	Guatemala
Argentina		El Salvador
		Nicaragua
		Costa Rica
		Panama
		Venezuela, R.B. de
		Colombia
		Ecuador
		Peru
		Paraguay
		Uruguay

Source: Original survey data.

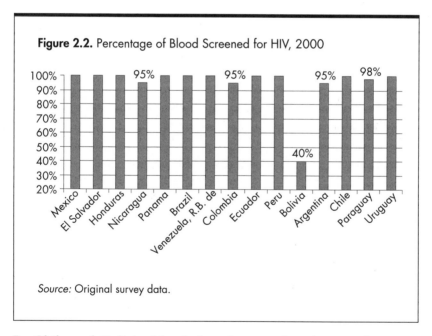

Figure 2.2. Percentage of Blood Screened for HIV, 2000

Source: Original survey data.

In Chile and Bolivia, blood donation was based on replacement donors (family members' donations for hospitalized patients), and in the other countries surveyed, altruistic donation coincided with other policies (table 2.14).

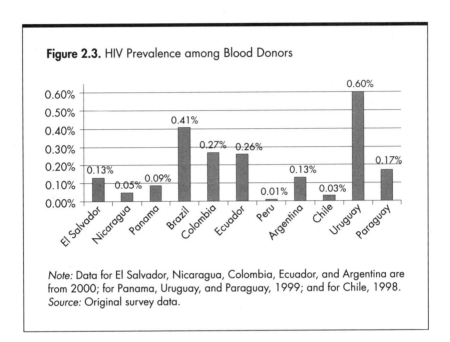

Figure 2.3. HIV Prevalence among Blood Donors

Note: Data for El Salvador, Nicaragua, Colombia, Ecuador, and Argentina are from 2000; for Panama, Uruguay, and Paraguay, 1999; and for Chile, 1998. *Source:* Original survey data.

Basic Needs for Improving the Epidemiological Surveillance of HIV/AIDS

All the survey respondents made reference to the need for increased resources for planning and consolidating the existing systems. The need for training and new technicians was a common theme. Regarding the information systems currently in place, respondents saw a need to improve the systems for reporting HIV/AIDS cases, especially in terms of ensuring their validity and comprehensiveness. Underreporting was one of the most common problems. Regarding sentinel surveillance, most of the problems related to the need for systematizing information systems and incorporating new subpopulations. According to some of those interviewed, second-generation surveillance is troublesome to those responsible for the surveillance systems, given the current lack of implementation and development in the region. In summary, the study concluded that increased resources, technically trained personnel, and political policy-related support are the primary objectives for improving HIV/AIDS surveillance in Latin America.

Conclusions: Strengths and Challenges

Strengths

- All countries developed epidemiological surveillance systems at the start of the epidemic.
- Allocation of resources and personnel has steadily increased since the 1980s.
- Surveillance systems with national coverage are in place.
- Information collection is coordinated with different actors (e.g., epidemiology offices, NGOs, universities, the military).
- Surveillance systems based on AIDS case notification are found to be well established through years of implementation.
- Human resources allocated to epidemiological surveillance have been extensive at the national level.
- Reporting of AIDS cases is mandatory.
- National standardized forms are available for HIV/AIDS case notification.
- Systems are in place for identification of duplicates.
- Most of the countries surveyed had structured schemes for sentinel surveillance of HIV integrated into the overall HIV information system.
- Some information on behavior is available through KAP studies.
- There are baseline studies on populations with high-risk behaviors.
- Surveillance plans have been developed for high-risk populations and behavior (ongoing or programmed).

- Almost all donated blood is screened, close to 100 percent in most countries.

- HIV testing is free or available at low cost in many countries.

- Epidemiological data are extensively and widely distributed.

- Evaluation of the surveillance system is carried out in most countries.

Challenges

- Persistent high levels of underreporting and delays in reporting remain. There is an urgent need to revise the procedures and circuits through which cases are reported.

- Gaps exist in human resources (e.g., technicians, training) at the local level.

- Case definition of HIV and AIDS varies greatly and probably warrants evaluation of the practicality and usefulness of some definitions in terms of availability of diagnostic tools and certain health centers' capacity.[1]

- HIV information systems are fed by a limited infrastructure of public laboratories and a diagnostic testing system that requires most populations to pay for their test and diagnosis.

- In some countries the confidentiality standards for HIV/AIDS reporting should be revised given the human rights and discrimination implications. Restricting access to case-identifying information to health care professionals who carry out the diagnosis and care of patients falls within the norms for professional conduct and should be considered a common goal.

- Methods for active surveillance are scarcely developed, especially in the countries most affected by the epidemic. Active surveillance could help reduce underreporting.

- Sentinel surveillance of HIV is neither systematized nor sufficiently developed. Most data are generated by periodic random studies that are not projected over time and lack evaluations of interventions or analysis of the epidemic, leaving authorities without the information necessary to make decisions.

- There are very few sentinel surveillance studies of the highest risk groups (MSM, CSWs, IDUs) and relatively more attention directed to the general population, which is more expensive to survey (due to the size of the population) and ultimately generates fewer prevention activities for the populations needing them most.

- Results of studies are poorly disseminated in scientific circles and are notably scarce at the international level.

- Little behavior surveillance takes place. Information is usually produced by periodic random studies, which are not always shared with HIV/AIDS programs. In some countries there are already plans for behavior surveillance, and results are expected in the next few years.

- In-depth evaluation of surveillance systems is needed. Often the supporting documents include descriptions of the process or reports on the status of the epidemic rather than a focus on the surveillance system.

- Study protocols vary widely, which makes it difficult to analyze the scope and trends of the epidemic. Furthermore, it leads to discrepancies in the results of different national or international studies.

- HIV information systems are fed by a limited infrastructure of public laboratories and a diagnostic testing system that requires most populations to pay for the test and diagnosis.

- Policies promoting HIV testing are lacking. This is a crucial element for increasing testing and diagnosis among high-risk populations, increasing counseling and prevention, and monitoring the epidemic. Testing is not always free or available in public centers, and sometimes there is limited access to anonymous diagnosis centers. Although these factors help regulate demand for the test, they have the negative consequence of reducing accessibility for those who need it.

- Blood safety policies are not as widespread as needed, although most countries screen at least 95 percent of blood. HIV prevalence among blood donors is still very high, while policies for exclusive voluntary and altruistic blood donation exist in only a few countries. Review and revision of blood safety policies would do much to improve these systems.

- Resources are needed for expanding epidemiological surveillance systems, training technicians, providing the necessary infrastructure for greater accessibility to testing and diagnosis, better implementing sentinel surveillance plans and registries, and providing systematic, secure treatment of epidemiological information.

- Political commitment is needed to strengthen and improve epidemiological surveillance.

Note

1. On the other hand, it is possible that health centers with various levels of infrastructure development would assign different sensitivity and predictive values to the same definition. This, in turn, would affect the validity and comprehensiveness of the records.

CHAPTER 3

National Responses to the Epidemic

Summary

The main objective of this chapter is to analyze and evaluate health sector capacity to fight the HIV/AIDS epidemic in Latin American countries. To this end, we consulted selected key respondents as part of our survey, including government officials, physicians, and non-governmental organization (NGO) representatives. National HIV/AIDS programs have different levels of development within ministries of health. However, they all have official identity and autonomy. Interinstitutional coordination and agreement are part of the national strategies.

HIV/AIDS prevention interventions have been numerous. Almost all the countries we surveyed carried out at least one mass media information campaign in 2000, and 57 percent confirmed that they had school-based HIV/AIDS prevention programs. Most recently, countries have carried out interventions focused on men who have sex with men (MSM), injecting drug users (IDUs), and prisoners. Coverage varies greatly. Programs targeted to commercial sex workers (CSWs) have the longest history.

Government responses to the injecting drug use epidemic have been insufficient. Few countries surveyed are implementing harm reduction programs, and coverage is sub par. Programs implemented by the NGOs surveyed have provided general information and prevention activities, and some have provided services and support to people living with HIV/AIDS (PLWHA). The target populations of the NGOs surveyed were primarily low-risk groups, while prisoners, MSM, CSWs, and IDUs received less attention. Ninety-four percent of NGOs indicated that homosexuality is discouraged in Latin America, highlighting the inherent challenge in providing services for MSM.

There is limited availability of HIV testing in public centers, and the high cost imposes barriers to both testing and counseling. Physician respondents confirmed that 67 percent of HIV-positive people did not seek health care until they were in advanced stages of infection or showed signs and symptoms of AIDS. The rate at which HIV testing is offered to pregnant women is very low, although this varies between countries. Antiretroviral therapy is provided to only half the patients who need it, and there is a significant percentage of PLWHA who lack resources for such treatment.

The main problems faced by national HIV/AIDS programs are political indecision on the part of government policymakers and lack of prioritization of the HIV/AIDS epidemic, which results in insufficient resource allocation. Physicians most often associated problems and barriers with insufficient government responses. NGOs attributed problems in controlling the epidemic to government policies, unmet needs in national program activities, and cultural and social values.

Introduction

The challenge of confronting HIV/AIDS in Latin America is a formidable one, requiring nothing less than the mobilization of many actors for the response. Over the past few years there have been continuous efforts to mobilize political leadership at the highest levels of national, regional, and global governance. A series of high-level events, including the United Nations General Assembly Special Session on

AIDS in June 2001, have resulted in HIV/AIDS now being recognized as a fundamental issue directly related to world development and security and requiring a truly global response. The World Bank has been one of the key advocates for expanding the response to HIV/AIDS and linking it more directly to development. Although this report focuses more on health sector–related issues, it is important to know and recognize the broader context in which the response to HIV/AIDS in Latin America is taking place.

At the country level, much has been achieved over the last few years. Efforts have focused on building political support for an effective national response to the epidemic. There have been important advocacy efforts to encourage national leaders to make a commitment to HIV/AIDS and build stronger multisectorial responses to the epidemic. Countries are developing national strategic plans or frameworks that spell out their national priorities regarding HIV/AIDS, and there has been a clear shift in the perception of the epidemic from a health-only to a broader social and developmental approach. The national strategic plan process also has contributed to stronger and more inclusive national coordination and partnership mechanisms with broad stakeholder representation.

Latin America and the Caribbean have made access to care available, more than anywhere in the developing world. Access to universal treatment with antiretroviral drugs has changed the response to HIV/AIDS in many countries.

Finally, achievements in coordination and regional responses (e.g., the creation of the Horizontal Technical Cooperation Group) as key pillars of intercountry collaboration should be acknowledged.

A comprehensive analysis of national responses to the epidemic would require a multisectorial analysis that goes beyond the intent of this study. This volume focuses on health sectors' national responses to the epidemic, and analyzes and evaluates the health sectors' capacity to fight the epidemic in Latin American countries through the eyes of key respondents involved in the prevention and control of the epidemic. These respondents include governments, through those responsible for national HIV/AIDS prevention and control programs, physicians working with HIV/AIDS, and NGOs working in the region. Our survey consulted the different actors through self-reported, semistructured questionnaires that were sent to the countries in advance and completed during face-to-face interviews by trained interviewers.

HIV/AIDS is an infectious disease transmitted from person to person through risk behaviors related to sexual practices (unprotected sex) and individual habits (sharing needles, syringes, or drug "works"), from mother to unborn child, or via unsafe practices and protocols (e.g., blood safety policies, clinical protocols). High-risk sexual behavior is the cause of most HIV cases in Latin America, followed by unsafe practices among IDUs (*HIV and AIDS in the Americas* 2001). This epidemic is a serious public developmental and health problem with significant repercussions in terms of morbidity and mortality, socioeconomic well-being, and the community in general. Therefore, its control and prevention require the participation and coordination of governments, civil society, and many other actors joining in a common multisectorial effort (World Bank 1997; United Nations Programme on HIV/AIDS [UNAIDS] 2000v; UNAIDS, the Prince of Wales Business Leaders Forum, and the Global Business Council on HIV and AIDS 2000).

National Agreements and Multisectorial Coordination

Most national HIV/AIDS prevention and control programs were created in the second half of the 1980s. Through the years, national programs have been shaped and reshaped, sometimes for the better, sometimes for the worse. Subsequently, some of the programs have grown and strengthened, while others have weakened due to political changes, decreased budgets, health sector reform, and other factors. National programs were established primarily under national ministries of health, specifically through the public health or epidemiology offices. Compared with other targeted health programs, national HIV/AIDS programs have had a different level of development and influence within ministries of health. Specifically, they have had more official identity and autonomy and have involved more multidisciplinary professionals. Governments have now declared AIDS a problem of the state, with the sole exception of those of the Andean region.

National Budgets for HIV/AIDS Control and Prevention

Our survey revealed that the Central American countries have the lowest budgets dedicated to HIV/AIDS in Latin America. There are marked differences in budget; notably, Argentina and Mexico spend more than US$1.00 per inhabitant, which is significantly more than other countries (table 3.1).

Table 3.1. Government Budgets for HIV/AIDS, 2000

COUNTRY OR SUBREGION	TOTAL BUDGET (US$)	BUDGET PER 100 INHABITANTS (US$)
Mexico	100,100,000	101.2
Central America		
Guatemala	641,025	5.6
El Salvador	—	—
Honduras	451,612	6.9
Nicaragua	100,000	1.9
Costa Rica	—	—
Panama	—	—
Brazil	—	—
Andean Region		
Venezuela, R.B. de	43,170	0.2
Colombia	250,000	0.6
Ecuador	—	—
Peru	5,150,000	20.0
Bolivia	—	—
Southern Cone		
Argentina	65,904,071	178.1
Paraguay	—	—
Uruguay	80,000	2.4
Chile	—	—

— Not available.
Source: Original survey data.

Multisectorial Coordination

Coordination and agreement among different government institutions and the civil society are essential for effective and efficient control of the epidemic (UNAIDS 1998), responding to national- and community-level needs. In Latin America, interinstitutional and civil coordination and agreement are part of national strategies.

Regarding intersectorial coordination, all countries[1] had collaboration agreements among the national program or ministry of health and other government administrations, regions, or states. In most countries, agreements had been signed with ministries of education, regions and municipalities, prisons, and national defense. The survey revealed that there were few activities coordinated with social service ministries, despite the fact that HIV/AIDS is a serious social issue (see table 3.2).

All countries except Panama and Paraguay had national committees for HIV/AIDS prevention and control interventions. These committees consisted of government and nongovernment participants involved in the fight against HIV/AIDS and provided a forum for consultation and evaluation (see table 3.3).

Community Responses: NGOs in Latin America

Findings from this survey indicate that in Latin America the number of HIV/AIDS-related NGOs per subregion varied substantially, from an average of 8.5 NGOs in Central America to 34 in the Andean Region and 60 in the Southern Cone. Brazil and Mexico had the most HIV/AIDS-related NGOs.

According to the national officials collaborating in this survey, only half the governments (Mexico, Honduras, Nicaragua, Brazil, Colombia, Argentina, and Chile) financed HIV/AIDS-related NGOs. This was corroborated by the NGOs surveyed; all did, indeed, confirm funding, with the exception of Honduras and Nicaragua (table 3.4).

Table 3.2. Collaboration between Ministries of Health and Other Government Institutions in the Fight against HIV/AIDS, 2000

COUNTRY OR SUBREGION	MINISTRY OF EDUCATION	MINISTRY OF DEFENSE	MINISTRY OF LABOR	MINISTRY OF SOCIAL AFFAIRS	PRISONS OR MINISTRY OF JUSTICE	DRUG PREVENTION INSTITUTION	REGIONS	MUNICIPALITIES
Mexico	✓					✓	✓	✓
Central America	83.3%	66.7%	33.3%	16.7%	83.3%		66.7%	66.7%
Guatemala	✓	✓			✓		✓	✓
El Salvador	✓	✓			✓		✓	✓
Honduras	✓	✓	✓		✓		✓	✓
Nicaragua	✓	✓	✓	✓	✓		✓	✓
Costa Rica	✓				✓			
Panama	—	—	—	—	—	—	—	—
Brazil	✓	✓	✓	✓	✓	✓	✓	✓
Andean Region	60.0%	20.0%	20.0%		40.0%		40.0%	40.0%
Venezuela, R.B. de	✓	✓			✓		✓	
Colombia	✓		✓		✓		✓	✓
Ecuador	✓							✓
Peru	—	—	—	—	—	—	—	—
Bolivia	—	—	—	—	—	—	—	—
Southern Cone	50.0%	50.0%	75.0%	50.0%	75.0%	75.0%	75.0%	75.0%
Argentina		✓	✓	✓	✓	✓	✓	✓
Paraguay	✓				✓		✓	
Uruguay	✓	✓	✓		✓	✓	✓	
Chile	✓	✓	✓	✓	✓	✓	✓	✓
Latin America	12 (70.5%)	8 (47.0%)	7 (41.2%)	4 (23.5%)	11 (64.7%)	5 (29.4%)	11 (64.7%)	11 (64.7%)

— Not available.

Note: Check marks indicate organizations that collaborate with the ministry of health in the fight against HIV. Blank cells indicate that the institution is not involved in the fight against HIV/AIDS.

Source: Original survey data.

88 • HIV/AIDS in Latin American Countries

Table 3.3. Countries with National Commissions for Evaluating HIV/AIDS Prevention and Control Activities, 2000

COUNTRY OR SUBREGION	NATIONAL EVALUATION COMMISSION
Mexico	✓
Central America	5
Guatemala	✓
El Salvador	✓
Honduras	✓
Nicaragua	✓
Costa Rica	✓
Panama	
Brazil	✓
Andean Region	3
Venezuela, R.B. de	✓
Colombia	✓
Ecuador	✓
Peru	
Bolivia	—
Southern Cone	3
Argentina	✓
Paraguay	
Uruguay	✓
Chile	✓
Latin America	13

— Not available.
Note: Blank cells indicate that the country does not have a national evaluation commission.
Source: Original survey data.

Table 3.4. Government Funding for HIV/AIDS-Related Nongovernmental Organizations, 2000

COUNTRY[a]	AMOUNT (US$)
Nicaragua	30,000
Honduras	104,000
Mexico	164,386
Argentina	880,506
Brazil	24,622,204
Colombia	Funds given, amount unknown
Chile	Funds given, amount unknown

a. No data were available from other countries.
Source: Original survey data.

Among the NGOs surveyed, 34.5 percent had received government funding within the last five years. Subregional differences were significant—in Brazil and Mexico all NGOs had received funds from the government, while in Central America, only 6.4 percent of financing came from the government.

The NGOs surveyed reported that when national programs allocated funds to NGOs, they were often targeted to the following populations: MSM, CSWs, PLWHA, and adolescents. NGOs in Guatemala, Mexico, and Uruguay stated that they received funding from other organizations, as well.

Relationship between NGOs and Governments

Besides financing, another way to estimate the level of coordination or collaboration between national or regional HIV/AIDS programs and NGOs is to calculate the frequency of institutional collaboration. This survey revealed that in Latin America overall, 67.5 percent of NGOs participated in evaluation committees, or groups that assess the activities of national programs. The number of meetings or contacts between NGOs and national programs in the past five years varied, but in almost every subregion, the NGOs surveyed had met with the national program more than twice (see table 3.5).

Despite scarce institutional incentives, a culture of providing dedicated, voluntary professional services for HIV/AIDS has arisen that has the voice and capacity to support its goals and beliefs through consultations with national programs and others.

HIV/AIDS Legislation

As a consequence of scientific and technical advances, and to protect human rights, countries have passed a significant amount of HIV/AIDS legislation. In some countries, there are extensive laws, rules, and norms; in most countries, legislation has mostly been passed regarding the safety and control of blood and blood products through systematic testing.

Table 3.5. Number and Percentage of NGOs Receiving Government Funding and Participating in National or Regional HIV/AIDS Program Evaluation Committees, 2000

COUNTRY OR SUBREGION	NGOs RECEIVING GOVERNMENT FUNDING	NGOs PARTICIPATING IN NATIONAL HIV/AIDS PROGRAM EVALUATION COMMITTEE
Mexico	5 (100.0%)	3 (60.0%)
Central America	2 (6.7%)	25 (83.3%)
Guatemala	1 (20.0%)	2 (40.0%)
El Salvador	1 (16.7%)	5 (83.3%)
Honduras	—	4 (100.0%)
Nicaragua	—	6 (100.0%)
Costa Rica	—	5 (100.0%)
Panama	—	3 (75.0%)
Brazil	5 (100.0%)	5 (100.0%)
Andean Region	7 (28.0%)	17 (68.0%)
Venezuela, R.B. de	1 (20.0%)	4 (80.0%)
Colombia	2 (50.0%)	2 (50.0%)
Ecuador	—	4 (80.0%)
Peru	4 (66.7%)	2 (33.3%)
Bolivia	—	5 (100.0%)
Southern Cone	10 (55.5%)	6 (33.3%)
Argentina	5 (100.0%)	3 (60.0%)
Paraguay	0	2 (50.0%)
Uruguay	2 (33.3%)	—
Chile	3 (100.0%)	1 (33.3%)
Latin America	29 (34.5%)	56 (67.5%)

— Not available.
Source: Original survey data.

Interventions for the General Population and Specific Groups

The government officials surveyed reported that in 2000 all the countries surveyed (except for Bolivia, Ecuador, and El Salvador, which did not provide data) carried out at least one mass media information campaign. Allocated budgets varied among countries. Some countries coordinated activities with World AIDS Day (Uruguay), Carnival celebrations (Panama), youth meetings (Honduras), or in association with specific geographic areas (Peru). The budget for these campaigns was highly variable among countries (table 3.6).

Table 3.6. Number and Budgets of Mass Media Campaigns, 2000

COUNTRY OR SUBREGION	NUMBER OF CAMPAIGNS	BUDGET FOR CAMPAIGNS (US$)
Mexico	1	109,375
Central America		
Guatemala	1	—
El Salvador	—	—
Honduras	3	18,900
Nicaragua	—	28,000
Costa Rica	1	—
Panama	1	—
Brazil	2	4,153,186
Andean Region		
Venezuela, R.B. de	1	2,000
Colombia	1	—
Ecuador	—	—
Peru	1	11,400
Bolivia	—	—
Southern Cone		
Argentina	6	90,000
Paraguay	4	15,285
Uruguay	1	10,000
Chile	1	—
Latin America (total)	24	4,438,146

— Not available.
Source: Original survey data.

According to data collected, in the past 10 years there have been few information campaigns for the general population. Brazil, Mexico, and some of the Central American countries ran these general campaigns most often (table 3.7).

Although sexual transmission is the most prevalent method of contracting HIV in all the countries, condom promotion as a central theme was reported by only a few of the campaigns carried out in the region.

Toll-free HIV/AIDS hotlines were widespread in the region and were most often run by NGOs; only Nicaragua and Ecuador did not provide this service, according to our survey data.

Table 3.7. Mass Media Campaigns Held from 1991 to 2000 for the General Population and Youths

COUNTRY	NUMBER OF CAMPAIGNS
Ecuador	None
Guatemala	1–3
Costa Rica	1–3
Peru	1–3
Argentina .	1–3
Colombia	3–5
Chile	3–5
Mexico	More than 5
El Salvador	More than 5
Honduras	More than 5
Nicaragua	More than 5
Brazil	More than 5
Venezuela, R.B. de	More than 5
Paraguay	More than 5
Uruguay	More than 5
Panama	—
Bolivia	—

— Not available.
Source: Original survey data.

Youths and Adolescents

Youths and adolescents constitute a large proportion of the Latin American population, and reaching these groups through school-based programs is one of the most effective interventions (UNAIDS 1997b; Merson, Dayton, and O'Reilly 2000; Centers for Disease Control and Prevention [CDC] 1999a). According to the respondents, in Latin America, school attendance by children 14 years and under was 76 percent, with the lowest percentages found in Central America and the Andean Region (see table 3.8).

In many countries, there is a significant proportion of children who do not attend school and who have an increased risk of contracting HIV through risky behavior possibly due to low educational level; they lack access to information through school-based education program, and they are hard to reach since they are not institutionalized.

Table 3.8. Percentage of Children up to 14 Years Attending School, 2000

COUNTRY[a]	%
Ecuador	30.6
Nicaragua	32.0
Honduras	64.0
Chile	87.0
Paraguay	91.0
Mexico	92.1
Brazil	95.7
Argentina	96.5
Uruguay	98.0
Average	76.3

a. No data were available for countries not listed.
Source: Original survey data.

This important group should be taken into account when planning youth-related activities.

According to the data collected through the survey, 62 percent of the countries had school-based HIV/AIDS prevention programs,* and 31 percent of the countries occasionally planned and provided such activities. Most school-based programs (64.3 percent) were designed and implemented in collaboration with the ministry of education (table 3.9).

Most respondents said that they could not identify budgets specifically allocated to these activities or the level of coverage of the school population. The information available shows that development of such activities is still lacking in schools for young people under 15 years of age.

High-risk adolescents have been the target of prevention interventions in half the countries, according to the respondents, although the exact groups and level of coverage varied. The amount invested in

---

*Here, "program" refers to an organized, systematized, and coherent group with integrated activities and services which are carried out with allocated resources and a goal of reaching previously determined objectives related to preventing new HIV infections in a defined population. This term does not refer to occasional activities, one-time activities or those which respond to an immediate, urgent demand.

Table 3.9. School-Based HIV/AIDS-Related Programs, 2000

COUNTRY OR SUBREGION	WITH SCHOOL-BASED PROGRAM	WITHOUT SCHOOL-BASED PROGRAM	OCCASIONAL ACTIVITIES
Mexico	✓		
Central America	3 (50.0%)	1 (16.7%)	2 (33.3%)
Guatemala		✓	
El Salvador	✓		
Honduras	✓		
Nicaragua	✓		
Costa Rica			✓
Panama			✓
Brazil	✓		
Andean Region	2 (50.0%)		2 (50.0%)
Venezuela, R.B. de	✓		
Colombia	✓		
Ecuador			✓
Peru			✓
Bolivia	—	—	—
Southern Cone	3 (66.7%)		1 (33.3%)
Argentina			✓
Paraguay	✓		
Uruguay	✓		
Chile	✓		
Latin America	10 (62.5%)	1 (6.2%)	5 (31.2%)

— Not available.
Source: Original survey data.

programs per adolescent varied (US$126 per adolescent in Honduras, US$27 in Brazil, US$25 in Uruguay, US$0.4 to US$3.0 in Paraguay, and an average of US$589 in Argentina). The majority of these programs were carried out by NGOs.

Men Who Have Sex with Men

All the countries surveyed, except Panama, had carried out interventions focused on MSM. Results from the survey indicate that in seven countries, these interventions were concrete programs and that in three countries such interventions were occasional, but steady. The most frequent interventions were information and education activities, workshops on safe sex, and counseling and condom distribution; many were planned and implemented through NGOs. The respondents indicated that these programs were very recent (beginning in 1999–2000) and that coverage varied greatly. This study could not identify the cost per beneficiary in the region as a whole either because records of beneficiaries and costs did not exist or because respondents were not aware of such information. However, during the study, it was found that in Honduras the cost per beneficiary of these programs was US$16, while in Mexico and Brazil it was US$1.

Male and Female Commercial Sex Workers

Data from this study show that 14 countries (82.3 percent) had programs targeting female CSWs, 12 countries (70 percent) had programs targeting male CSWs, and 11 countries (65 percent) had programs targeting transvestites (table 3.10). These programs had the

Table 3.10. Countries with HIV/AIDS Programs Focused on Commercial Sex Workers, 2000

COUNTRY OR SUBREGION	WOMEN	MEN	TRANSVESTITES
Mexico	yes	yes	—
Central America			
Guatemala	yes	yes	yes
El Salvador	yes	yes	yes
Honduras	yes	yes	yes
Nicaragua	yes	yes	yes
Costa Rica	no	no	no
Panama	no	no	no
Brazil	yes	yes	yes
Andean Region			
Venezuela, R.B. de	yes	yes	yes
Colombia	yes	yes	yes
Ecuador	yes	no	no
Peru	yes	yes	yes
Bolivia	—	—	—
Southern Cone			
Argentina	yes	yes	yes
Paraguay	yes	yes	no
Uruguay	yes	yes	yes
Chile	yes	no	yes

— Not available.
Source: Original survey data.

most historical background, dating to the 1990s; however, systematized organization and data collection did not begin until recently (1999–2000). Respondents indicated that most interventions involved distribution of educational materials, counseling, and promotion of peer training.

Access to health care services is a basic need for controlling the disease from the clinical point of view, both to provide early diagnosis and treatment of HIV and to promote preventive measures in high-risk populations such as CSWs (Ghys and others 2001; Levine and others 1998). The survey data revealed that in 59 percent of the countries, health care services were free for CSWs. In Mexico, Peru, and Uruguay, for example, there were services specifically designed and reserved for CSWs, while in Ecuador such health care was provided through NGOs.

Injecting Drug Users

Injecting drug use is most prevalent in Mexico, Brazil, and the Southern Cone; respondents from other countries reported that other methods of drug use (e.g., inhalants, pills) were more common. There are few estimates published of the size of the IDU population in each country. According to survey respondents, Chile had 29,046 IDUs, Mexico had 48,000, and Argentina had 64,558.

The most commonly injected drug was cocaine (reported in 71.4 percent of countries); only Mexico and Colombia reported higher rates of IV heroin use (Hudgins, McCusker, and Stoddard 1995).

According to the respondents, government responses to the IV drug use epidemic had been insufficient, and very few countries were implementing harm reduction programs, which often offered sub-par coverage. Seven countries either had no program or had only sporadic "drug-free" programs that were barely effective for harm reduction and HIV control purposes (Des Jarlais 1995; Drucker and others 1998; see table 3.11). Most interventions for IDUs consisted of needle exchange programs (in which used needles can be exchanged for sterile ones) and training on how to better clean their instruments.[3] The data provided for the study were not precise, and

Table 3.11. Availability of Interventions for Injecting Drug Users, 2000

COUNTRY OR SUBREGION	DRUG-FREE OR DRUG PREVENTION PROGRAMS	HARM REDUCTION PROGRAMS
Mexico	✓	✓
Central America		
Guatemala	✓	
El Salvador	✓	
Honduras	—	—
Nicaragua	✓	✓
Costa Rica	—	—
Panama	—	—
Brazil	✓	✓
Andean Region		
Venezuela, R.B. de	—	—
Colombia		✓
Ecuador	—	—
Peru	—	—
Bolivia		
Southern Cone		
Argentina	✓	✓
Paraguay		
Uruguay	✓	
Chile	✓	✓

— Not available.
Note: Blank cells indicate that there are no interventions for injecting drug users.
Source: Original survey data.

few data were available on the beneficiaries or budgets in all countries. In the case of Brazil, it can be estimated that needle exchange programs cost US$24,000 each, and the cost per IDU was as high as US$18. Overall, the study concluded that needle exchange programs and other harm reduction methods in Latin America were scarce and, with the exception of Brazil, were insufficient when considering the scope of the HIV/AIDS epidemic and its relation to injecting drug use.

Survey data revealed that clinical attention to drug users is scarce in Latin America (table 3.12). Even countries like Mexico, Argentina, and Chile had insufficient infrastructures and resources for effectively treating this population. Aside from national drug prevention, control, and treatment programs, the groups most involved in fighting drug use were the few independent centers caring for drug addicts and

98 • HIV/AIDS in Latin American Countries

Table 3.12. Availability of Centers Specialized in Treatment of Injecting Drug Users, 2000

COUNTRY	NUMBER OF CENTERS
Mexico	1
El Salvador	1
Nicaragua	8
Costa Rica	1
Panama	1
Brazil	26
Peru	1
Paraguay	7
Uruguay	1

Source: Original survey data.

drug-related NGOs. According to the respondents, health professionals and pharmacists were rarely involved in treating this population.

Prisoners

The rate of HIV infection among prisoners varied from country to country. Often, countries with the highest prevalence rates among prisoners also had the highest rates among IDUs. In some countries the rates reported among prisoners were alarmingly high (e.g., El Salvador), although it can be presumed that the highest prevalence rates among prisoners (based on rates among IDUs) would be found in the Southern Cone and Brazil (figure 3.1).

Survey respondents from 13 countries (76.5 percent) stated that they had HIV prevention programs for prisoners; Honduras and several countries of the Andean Region did not have such programs (see table 3.13). According to the information collected, in Central America these programs began recently (1999–2000) and consisted primarily of health education and educational material distribution. Coverage was scarce, and interventions were sporadic. In Mexico, these programs began earlier in the 1990s and provided a wide range of services, although coverage was still low. Programs offered in Mexico included HIV testing, condom distribution, and distribution

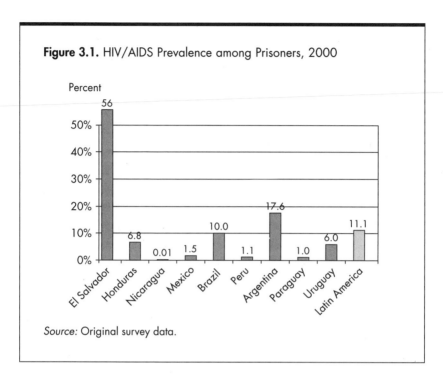

Figure 3.1. HIV/AIDS Prevalence among Prisoners, 2000

Source: Original survey data.

of sterile supplies for injecting drug use. Brazil also offered many services to a large number of prisoners. Recently, Southern Cone countries (e.g., Argentina in 1999) began implementing a wide variety of prevention services that were more prevalent in prisons in the larger cities. Overall, prisoners lacked sterile supplies and permanent access to condoms since distribution was sporadic. There were no data available on health care for prisoners with HIV, and there was also a gap in information on the coordination of services within and outside prisons for preventing, controlling, and treating HIV within prisons.

Outreach Programs for Hard-to-Reach Populations

The goal of outreach programs is to establish contacts with people with high or moderate risk for contracting HIV. Specifically, these programs should be managed to drive people to health care and prevention services, to compile information needed to protect these populations from HIV, and to provide social or emotional support

Table 3.13. HIV Prevention Programs in Prisons, 2000

COUNTRY OR SUBREGION	HIV PREVENTION PROGRAMS
Mexico	✓
Central America	5
Guatemala	✓
El Salvador	✓
Honduras	
Nicaragua	✓
Costa Rica	✓
Panama	✓
Brazil	✓
Andean Region	2
Venezuela, R.B. de	
Colombia	✓
Ecuador	
Peru	✓
Bolivia	
Southern Cone	4
Argentina	✓
Paraguay	✓
Uruguay	✓
Chile	✓
Latin America	13

Note: Blank cells indicate that the country does not have HIV prevention programs in its prisons.
Source: Original survey data.

(National Institute on Drug Abuse 2000; Trotter, Bowen, and Potter 1995; Krieger and others 1999). Many of these high-risk, hard-to-reach populations (e.g., CSWs, IDUs, marginalized groups) are accessible only through such programs. The data collected show that with the exception of Brazil and Mexico, outreach programs were scarce in the region (table 3.14).

NGOs' Contributions to HIV/AIDS Control in Latin America

NGOs in the region had different goals and covered a wide range of needs, including information and prevention and psychological, social, and family support for those affected. More than half of NGO

Table 3.14. HIV/AIDS Outreach Programs, 2000

COUNTRY OR SUBREGION[a]	OUTREACH PROGRAMS AVAILABLE			
	IDUs	MSM	CSWs	HIGH-RISK ADOLESCENTS
Mexico	✓	✓	✓	✓
Central America	0	1	1	1
Guatemala	no	✓	✓	✓
Brazil	✓	✓	✓	✓
Andean Region	1	1	1	0
Colombia	✓	✓	✓	no
Southern Cone	2	3	1	2
Argentina	✓	✓		
Paraguay		✓		✓
Uruguay	✓	✓	✓	✓
Latin America	5	7	5	5

a. Countries not listed do not have outreach programs.
Note: CSW = commercial sex worker; IDU = injecting drug user; MSM = men who have sex with men.
Source: Original survey data.

respondents confirmed that they provided these services. There were few NGOs with one single purpose; rather, it was more common for NGOs to provide a number of different HIV/AIDS-related services.

A review of the programs implemented by the NGOs surveyed (366 programs[*] by a total of 84 NGOs surveyed) shows that a little over half were involved in general information and prevention activities, including printing educational materials, and the rest provided services and support to PLWHA (figure 3.2).

Among these 366 programs, 215 were focused on targeted populations. As shown in figure 3.3, half of these programs were for women and adolescents, and the rest were for groups at high risk of contracting HIV.

---

[*]"Program" refers to an organized, systematized, and coherent group with integrated activities and services which are carried out with allocated resources and a goal of reaching previously determined objectives. This term does not refer to occasional activities, one-time activities or those that respond to an immediate, urgent demand.

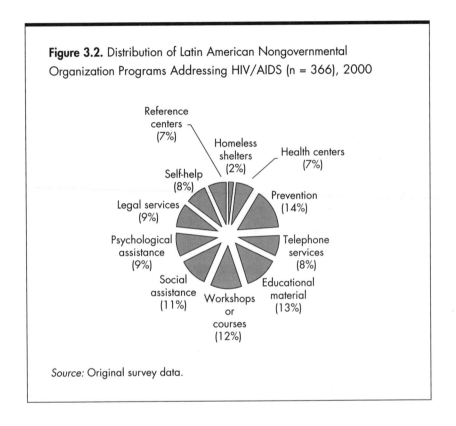

Figure 3.2. Distribution of Latin American Nongovernmental Organization Programs Addressing HIV/AIDS (n = 366), 2000

Reference centers (7%)

Homeless shelters (2%)

Health centers (7%)

Self-help (8%)

Prevention (14%)

Legal services (9%)

Psychological assistance (9%)

Telephone services (8%)

Social assistance (11%)

Educational material (13%)

Workshops or courses (12%)

Source: Original survey data.

The populations targeted included youths (70.2 percent), women (54.7 percent), MSM (48.8 percent), and CSWs (46.4 percent). Although prisoners and IDUs are at high risk of contracting HIV, they did not receive much attention from NGOs. This is particularly alarming in the Southern Cone, where HIV prevalence among these populations is very high.

Beneficiaries and Costs of the Programs Under Way

There were many difficulties in collecting information regarding NGOs' population coverage and budgets since, in most cases, the people completing the questionnaires for this study were more involved in the design and implementation of programs than collecting and maintaining such data. Few NGO respondents could

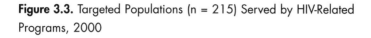

Figure 3.3. Targeted Populations (n = 215) Served by HIV-Related Programs, 2000

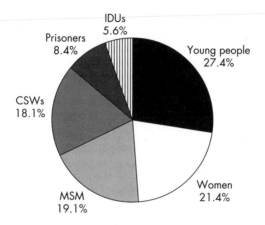

Note: CSW = commercial sex worker; IDU = injecting drug user; MSM = men who have sex with men.
Source: Original survey data.

identify the number of beneficiaries for each program, and information on budgets for each activity was limited since NGOs do not always maintain this information. Consequently, the data presented in figures 3.4 and 3.5 reflect only the responses of NGOs that had this information. It can be assumed that the actual number of beneficiaries and costs were higher than those presented.

Overall, programs for PLWHA, particularly hospices (US$606 per beneficiary), were most costly, followed by social support (US$108 per beneficiary). Costs varied among subregions, depending on the level of volunteer contributions and systems for contracting or payment of services for employees. From an economic point of view, programs providing support for PLWHA and self-supported programs were the most efficient. Costs per beneficiary for such programs were relatively similar among subregions except for Brazil, where the cost was higher (US$66.3 per beneficiary).

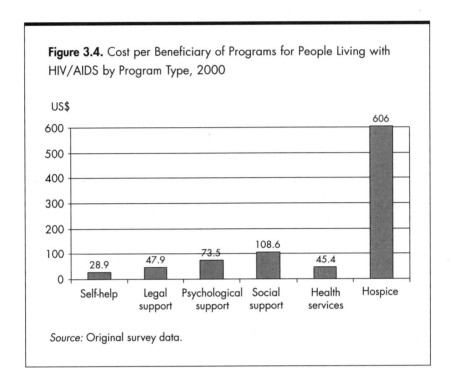

Figure 3.4. Cost per Beneficiary of Programs for People Living with HIV/AIDS by Program Type, 2000

Source: Original survey data.

Our data show that except for prisoners, programs targeting specific populations had an average cost of US$10 to US$20 per person. CSW programs were the least expensive, averaging US$10 per beneficiary, except in the case of Brazil, where the cost was higher. Programs for MSM cost about US$20 per person; this high average was largely due to the high costs found in Brazil and the Southern Cone. Youth- and women-based programs were the most expensive, yet it is important to keep in mind the large number of at-risk beneficiaries found in these population subgroups. The highest costs per beneficiary were found in Brazil and Central America (for women-targeted programs) and Mexico (for youth programs).

The most economical interventions were information dissemination and prevention programs, such as the toll-free HIV/AIDS information and support hotlines that offered wide coverage at a very low cost (US$2 per person). With the exception of the Southern Cone,

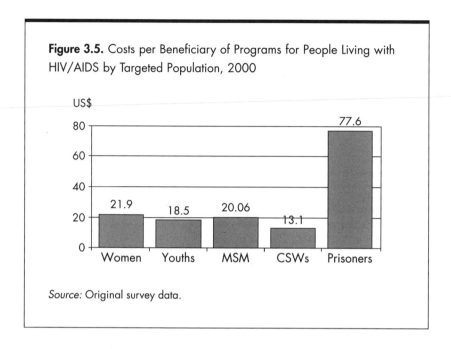

Figure 3.5. Costs per Beneficiary of Programs for People Living with HIV/AIDS by Targeted Population, 2000

Source: Original survey data.

information and prevention programs, including the printing of instructional materials, were very low cost activities.

Cost-Effectiveness: The Big Question

Measuring the costs of existing HIV/AIDS prevention programs per person reached is an essential part of developing the appropriate strategies for scaling up and program planning, but much of this essential information for priority setting remains elusive. To obtain the greatest benefit from a fixed budget, policy makers and program managers require information about the cost *per infection averted* or per life-year saved. This information typically is expressed in terms of the cost-effectiveness ratio, in which the numerator represents the net cost (e.g., the cost of condom distribution plus dissemination of appropriate educational messages minus the treatment and other costs not incurred because of the beneficial effects of the intervention) over the desired health outcome, such as the reduction of illness or death from HIV/AIDS. In concept, if this ratio is calculated for all interventions competing for common resources, decision makers can assign resources on the basis of cost-effectiveness, maximizing the good (i.e., lives saved) obtained from a given budget.

Estimating cost-effectiveness is difficult in all health care disciplines, but HIV/AIDS interventions represent a particularly daunting challenge. Decomposing the elements of the cost-effectiveness ratio—costs of the interventions, costs not incurred because of the intervention, and effectiveness of the intervention—demonstrates the complexity of this analysis.

Costs of HIV/AIDS prevention strategies are difficult to calculate, largely because they tend to depend on hard-to-quantify outreach strategies, peer counselors, and expansion of existing NGO activities. Often, there are no clear protocols for prevention activities; they evolve in an idiosyncratic manner, and service statistics are often exaggerated. In addition, we face a question about the perspective from which the costs are calculated—do we care about all social costs implied by an intervention, or just the costs to the provider? Although these issues complicate the cost estimates, it is possible to arrive at credible per person estimates of costs.

Estimating the savings in treatment averted as a result of the interventions carried out is a huge undertaking, typically requiring assumptions. Analysts must make "best guess" estimates about the effectiveness of the interventions being assessed—for example, out of 1,000 people reached with condoms and education, one infection per year is averted— and then must estimate the potential per case costs associated with the treatment of opportunistic infections and other ailments affecting PLWHA. These treatment costs depend largely on the characteristics and underlying cost structure of the health care system, as well as accepted treatment protocols, which have changed rapidly over time and are likely to continue to evolve with scientific discovery and technological innovation.

Estimates of the infections averted or the disability-adjusted life years saved by the intervention, which constitute the denominator of the cost-effectiveness ratio, also require strong assumptions. To further complicate matters, we are faced with the question of whether to include in the "effectiveness" estimate only the effect on the population directly benefiting from the intervention, or whether to consider the infections averted because of the reduced prevalence of HIV in the population—that is, the secondary, tertiary, and other future infections prevented because of the reduction in the number of infections in the population directly targeted. With HIV/AIDS, as with any infectious disease, the multiplier effect of preventive activities can be many times larger than the direct effects, depending on the rate of spread of the disease in the population, which itself depends on a number of underlying epidemiological, demographic, and social characteristics. In short, viewing the effects of preventive activities in a dynamic fashion is critical to arriving at a true picture of the benefits of prevention, but this is a complex empirical task.

With all these methodological complications, is there any point in attempting estimates of cost-effectiveness? The question can be answered only by considering the alternative: allocating scarce health care resources on the basis of allocation rules or practices that do not consider the quantity of the benefits per dollar spent. For example, a budget could be allocated on the basis of beliefs about the worthiness or "innocence" of the beneficiary populations (e.g., more for babies affected by mother-to-child transmission than for MSM, who are assumed by some to have brought the disease upon themselves), or on the basis of the political influence of the organizations receiving funding, or even across beneficiary populations in a way that is proportional to the estimated prevalence of the disease across those populations (a common strategy intended to achieve "fairness"). While each of these approaches to resource allocation has its advocates, none is likely to lead to the greatest number of HIV infections averted per dollar spent—arguably the essential objective underlying all HIV/AIDS prevention programs. Only the application of cost-effectiveness analysis—with all its difficulties and imperfections—will lead to this outcome.

A number of studies have been conducted to develop best guess estimates of the cost-effectiveness of specific interventions, but most of the evidence comes from industrialized countries. Jha and others (2001) compared the efficiency ratio, effect size, and cost-effectiveness of different evidenced-based interventions for HIV prevention for developing countries. Their findings show that interventions for CSWs have the lowest cost per infection averted ($8–$12), followed by sexually transmitted infection (STI) management interventions ($218), voluntary counseling and testing ($249–$346), and antiretroviral therapy for HIV-positive pregnant women ($276).

Prevention resources should be allocated to prevent as many infections as possible. Such an allocation must consider the cost and effectiveness of programs, as well as estimates of HIV incidence (UNAIDS 2000n), to allocate the right amount of money to programs for each specific risk group. A follow-up World Bank study will attempt to undertake exactly this approach and determine appropriate ways of allocating limited HIV/AIDS prevention resources among programs for different population groups (box 3.1).

The Population's Level of Knowledge of Transmission Methods and Prevention

Most of the answers to the survey confirmed that countries had carried out knowledge, attitude, and practice (KAP) surveys regarding HIV/AIDS, either through ministries of health or other institutions or agencies, in order to determine the population's level of knowledge regarding HIV/AIDS. Unfortunately, the results and lessons from these studies have not been shared with a wide audience and have barely been used to guide decision making in national programs.

Based on responses from the physicians participating in the survey, 20 percent of people would have a good level of knowledge, 66 percent would have some knowledge, and 14 percent would have little or no knowledge of modes of transmission and prevention of HIV/AIDS.

Social Attitudes Toward Sexual Orientation

The proved increased risk of contracting HIV through unprotected anal intercourse has resulted in categorizing MSM, and other groups

Box 3.1. Toward More Rational Allocation Decisions

Over the next few months, the World Bank proposes to pilot test, in one Central American country, a methodology to determine the allocation of resources among prevention interventions that maximizes the number of infections averted. The exercise will draw on the techniques elaborated in *No Time to Lose* (Ruiz and others 2000) and relies on subjective and systematic construction of two sets of estimates: one related to the epidemiology of HIV (i.e., new infections in the target populations) and one related to program effectiveness (i.e., new infections prevented at different levels of program funding) by subgroup. The elaboration of these variables relies heavily on consensus among local and international experts.

It is expected that this exercise will inform policy decisions by explicitly illustrating the opportunity cost of alternative allocation mechanisms (e.g., based on prevalence or on number of AIDS cases). The exercise may also generate renewed policy interest in tracking incidence and program effectiveness, because doing so would dramatically improve allocation decisions and revert the epidemic faster.

with this practice, as high risk since the beginning of the epidemic (UNAIDS 2000a; Catania and others 2001; McFarland and Cáceres 2001). This risk factor leads to the need for prevention interventions and health and social services specifically targeted to this population. Intolerant social attitudes, or homophobia, are not only human rights infringements; such attitudes impede effective prevention, early diagnosis, and appropriate treatment for this group. Participating NGOs were asked about the sociocultural attitudes regarding homosexuality and if there were any laws or regulations that restricted or prohibited homosexual orientation (table 3.15). Ninety-four percent of the NGOs surveyed indicated that homosexuality is discouraged in Latin America, either through sociocultural attitudes (57.8 percent) or sociocultural attitudes combined with legal penalties (36.1 percent). In Mexico and Brazil, most NGOs indicated that the restrictions are

Table 3.15. Percentage of NGOs Surveyed That Identified Homosexuality Restrictions, 2000 (n = 83)

COUNTRY OR SUBREGION	RESTRICTIONS ON HOMOSEXUALITY		
	SOCIOCULTURAL	NONE	SOCIOCULTURAL AND LEGAL
Mexico	40.0	—	60.0
Central America	51.6	9.7	38.7
Guatemala	50.0	16.7	33.3
El Salvador	83.3	—	16.7
Honduras	75.0	—	25.0
Nicaragua	—	16.7	83.3
Costa Rica	60.0	20.0	20.0
Panama	50.0	—	50.0
Brazil	20.0	—	80.0
Andean Region	68.0	4.0	28.0
Venezuela, R.B. de	60.0	—	40.0
Colombia	50.0	25.0	25.0
Ecuador	80.0	—	20.0
Peru	66.7	—	33.3
Bolivia	80.0	—	20.0
Southern Cone	70.6	5.9	23.5
Argentina	60.0	—	40.0
Paraguay	75.0	25.0	—
Uruguay	83.3	—	16.7
Chile	50.0	—	50.0
Latin America	57.8	6.1	36.1

— Not available.
Source: Original survey data.

both sociocultural (80 percent) and legal (60 percent), although specific laws mandating penalization were not identified. Thirty-eight percent of NGOs in Central America claimed that combined sociocultural and legal restrictions are the main prohibitive factors; in Nicaragua five NGOs mentioned penalizations for homosexuality, and in Guatemala punitive legislation was cited, although a specific law was not identified (see table 3.16).

HIV Infection Rates in High-Risk Populations

Data obtained from national programs on the number of HIV tests carried out in 2000 are not consistent with data obtained from the

Table 3.16. Legal Restrictions on Homosexuality

COUNTRY	TYPES OF LEGAL RESTRICTIONS
Mexico	Subject to "police repression as an illegal activity" (according to one NGO).
Guatemala	There are some gaps in the legislation, but there are punitive repercussions (according to one NGO). Special legal restrictions exist against transvestites (according to one NGO).
Nicaragua	Penalties according to Law 150, article 204 (cited by four NGOs).
Costa Rica	Legal restrictions exist. The general law for treatment of AIDS is not generally followed (according to one NGO).
Brazil	Couples are not legally recognized; therefore, couples may not share benefits or adopt children (cited by three NGOs).
Argentina	Subject to involvement of law enforcement officials and imprisonment. The law does not permit homosexual couples, and there are edicts and police norms against homosexual behavior.
Peru	Formal marriage is not allowed, and inheritance of goods and money and adoption are prohibited.
Uruguay	Legal restrictions exist. Couples are not legally recognized and are not mentioned in family rights laws.
El Salvador, Honduras, Panama, Venezuela, R.B. de, Colombia, Ecuador, Bolivia, Chile	No response was provided on the questionnaire.

Note: NGO = nongovernmental organization.
Source: Original survey data.

epidemiological surveillance offices (except in the República Bolivariana de Venezuela and Nicaragua). The same inconsistency was found in data regarding the prevalence rates in high-risk populations; only Mexico and Honduras provided data that were consistent among various sources (see table 3.17). These inconsistencies point to a lack of communication between national programs and epidemiological surveillance offices.

Table 3.17. HIV Prevalence among High-Risk Populations and Pregnant Women, 2000

COUNTRY OR SUBREGION	NUMBER OF HIV TESTS CONDUCTED	NUMBER OF IDUs TREATED	HIV PREVALANCE IN IDUs	HIV PREVALENCE IN MSM	HIV PREVALANCE IN CSWs	HIV PREVALANCE IN PREGNANT WOMEN
Mexico	251,763	800	4.60	15.00	0.35	0.09
Central America						
Guatemala	4,000	—	—	—	—	—
El Salvador	—	—	—	—	—	1.4
Honduras	—	—	—	8.0	9.9	0.7
Nicaragua	50,000	—	—	35.0	2.0	—
Costa Rica	—	—	—	—	—	0.9
Panama	93,500	—	—	—	—	0.5
Brazil	—	—	37.0	8.9	7.0	—
Andean Region						
Venezuela, R.B. de	200,000	—	—	70.0	—	0.01
Colombia	—	—	—	18.9	0.1	<1
Ecuador	—	—	—	11.3	0.6	0.3
Peru	—	—	—	11.0	1.2	0.0
Bolivia	—	—	—	0.04	0.03	0.0
Southern Cone						
Argentina	800,000	1,000	45.9	14.9	1.7	0.7
Paraguay	—	—	—	—	—	—
Uruguay	—	—	25.0	21.0	0.4	0.3
Chile	—	—	—	—	—	0.05

— Not available.

Note: CSW = commercial sex workers; IDU = injecting drug user; MSM = men who have sex with men.

Source: Original survey data.

Table 3.18. Number of Condoms Distributed by Ministries of Health and Budgets, 2000

COUNTRY[a]	NUMBER OF CONDOMS FINANCED	BUDGET FOR CONDOMS (US$)
Mexico	—	2,500,000
Honduras	300,000	10,000
Nicaragua	5,000,000	—
Brazil	200,000,000	6,000,000
Venezuela, R.B. de	2,000,000	—
Colombia	—	18,000
Peru	11,000,000	11,600,000
Argentina	200,000	20,000
Uruguay	—	20,000
Chile	1,000,000	59,000

— Not available.
a. Countries not listed do not distribute condoms.
Source: Original survey data.

Condom Distribution

According to the National HIV/AIDS programs surveyed, 59 percent of the countries financed condom distribution in 2000. Regionally, US$20.2 million financed the distribution of 219.5 million condoms. The unit cost per condom was about US$0.09 (table 3.18). Most often, condoms were distributed to zones where CSWs work, areas frequented by MSM, pharmacies, and NGOs. Colleges and universities did not receive government-provided condoms.

Quality control is important not only to prevent disease transmission, but also to maintain consumer satisfaction and confidence, which are crucial for encouraging safe sex behavior. Only half the countries had norms regulating condom quality; in the Andean Region, condom quality control is largely nonexistent, according to the data collected.

Prevention of Mother-to-Child Transmission

The availability of highly active antiretrovirals, prophylaxis with AZT, and new recommendations for labor and delivery for HIV-positive pregnant women have resulted in a significant decrease in mother-to-child transmission of HIV (UNAIDS 1999a, 1999b; CDC 2001b; International Perinatal HIV Group 1999). However, these achievements are possible only through early and efficient diagnosis of pregnant women. For this reason, it is important to offer HIV testing to pregnant women and to ensure easy access to diagnosis and treatment services.

Seven countries (Brazil, Honduras, Costa Rica, Peru, República Bolivariana de Venezuela, Argentina, and Uruguay) confirmed that they had protocols for offering the HIV test to all pregnant women, although the actual coverage in terms of numbers of tests offered varied between countries. For instance, Honduras had one of the highest prevalence rates in Central America, and yet according to the respondents, it offered HIV testing to only 8.7 percent of pregnant women (figure 3.6). Access to antiretroviral prophylaxis was also very low (only 20 percent in Honduras and 40 percent in Brazil), with substantial differences between subregions (see figure 3.7), which is unfortunate since such prophylactic measures are one of the simplest and most effective ways to prevent HIV transmission.

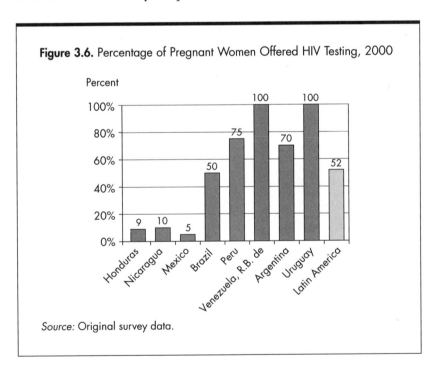

Figure 3.6. Percentage of Pregnant Women Offered HIV Testing, 2000

Source: Original survey data.

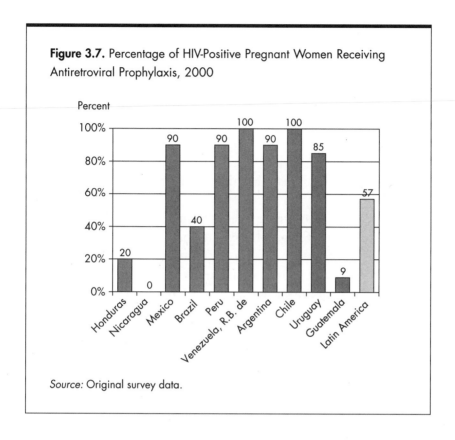

Figure 3.7. Percentage of HIV-Positive Pregnant Women Receiving Antiretroviral Prophylaxis, 2000

Source: Original survey data.

Health and Social Services

Access to Health Services and Prevention Interventions for High-Risk Populations

Information provided for this study about health centers, STI diagnosis and treatment centers, and hospitals with programs specifically for HIV/AIDS (testing, counseling, condom distribution, health education) differed greatly among countries and subregions, and there was a tendency to overestimate services provided. In general, national programs interviewed confirmed that almost all health centers (STI centers, primary care centers, and hospitals) had prevention programs planned specifically for HIV/AIDS, including voluntary testing and counseling, health education, and condom distribution. Information provided by physicians and NGOs regarding coverage and access to health services differed greatly from that provided by governments. In general, the government respondents saw access to health services as being wider than did physicians and as much wider than did NGO respondents.

Availability of Clinical Practice Guidelines

According to respondents, clinical practice guidelines for HIV/AIDS patients (measured by current knowledge and availability of resources) were scarce. In areas where access to antiretrovirals was limited, national guidelines for prophylaxis against opportunistic infections were also lacking or were rarely used (only 15.6 percent of countries). Forty-three percent of physicians surveyed stated that they had formal guidelines for managing antiretrovirals but that such guidelines were scarcely distributed or not well known in subregions such as the Andean Region and the Southern Cone (28.5 percent and 35.7 percent, respectively). Several physicians announced that new guidelines would soon be available, and many others usually consulted guidelines from international organizations (table 3.19).

According to responses from national program directors, health services, other than antiretroviral therapy, were free and universally offered in six countries (Costa Rica, Brazil, República Bolivariana de Venezuela, Argentina, Chile, and Paraguay). In six other countries (Honduras, Nicaragua, Panama, Peru, Colombia, and Mexico) health services were provided to people with insurance, and in the rest of Latin America such services were paid by the patient out of pocket. Often, ministries of health provided "welfare" services, but coverage was scarce and infrastructure and resources very limited. With few exceptions, a very small part of the population was covered by social security, especially in Central American countries.

Access to HIV Testing

Physicians and NGOs that were surveyed had similar estimates regarding conditions related to access to HIV testing. Fifty-one percent of

Table 3.19. Percentage of Physicians Surveyed (n = 64) Confirming Availability of Guidelines for Clinical Management and Treatment of PLWHA, 2000

COUNTRY OR SUBREGION	FULL MANAGEMENT	ARV THERAPY	PREVENTION OF MOTHER-TO-CHILD TRANSMISSION	PREVENTION OF OPPORTUNISTIC INFECTIONS
Mexico	20.0	80.0	none	40.0
Central America	15.8	47.3	15.7	21.1
Guatemala	none	33.3	none	33.3
El Salvador	40.0	40.0	none	20.0
Honduras	33.3	33.3	none	33.3
Nicaragua	none	none	none	none
Costa Rica	none	100.0	75.0	25.0
Panama	none	50.0	none	none
Brazil	none	80.0	none	none
Andean Region	9.5	28.5	none	19.0
Venezuela, R.B. de	none	66.6	none	25.0
Colombia	none	none	none	none
Ecuador	25.0	25.0	none	none
Peru	none	60.0	none	60.0
Bolivia	33.0	none	none	none
Southern Cone	7.1	35.7	14.3	none
Argentina	20.0	60.0	40.0	none
Paraguay	none	none	none	none
Uruguay	none	none	none	none
Chile	none	66.7	none	none
Latin America	10.9	43.7	7.8	15.6

Note: None = no guidelines exist. ARV = antiretroviral; PLWHA = people living with HIV/AIDS.
Source: Original survey data.

physicians and 54 percent of NGOs felt that HIV testing was available to the population. According to physicians, the average cost of the test in public health centers was US$21 and US$56 in private centers. There were few differences among subregions in terms of cost in public centers; however, there was a wide range of prices for testing in private centers—from US$49 in Central America to more than US$100 in Mexico (see table 3.20).

According to the participating NGOs, the main barrier to testing in all subregions and countries was social discrimination, followed by low demand for the test in high-risk populations and the infrequency of offering voluntary testing in health centers. In the Andean Region,

Table 3.20. Average Cost of HIV Testing in Public and Private Health Centers, 2000 (US$)

COUNTRY OR SUBREGION	COST IN PUBLIC HEALTH CENTERS (n = 22)	COST IN PRIVATE HEALTH CENTERS (n = 46)
Mexico	19.0	106.0
Central America (average)	15.6	49.0
Guatemala	5.0	71.3
El Salvador	18.7	58.3
Honduras	—	35.0
Nicaragua	10.0	15.0
Costa Rica	35.0	—
Panama	14.0	32.5
Brazil	free	32.5
Andean Region (average)	25.4	54.3
Venezuela	82.0	95.0
Colombia	10.0	40.0
Ecuador	43.0	25.3
Peru	23.4	74.2
Bolivia	8.5	23.7
Southern Cone (average)	—	50.2
Argentina	—	112.5
Paraguay	—	25.0
Uruguay	—	5.7
Chile	—	10.0
Latin America (average)	20.9	56.7

— Not available.
Source: Original survey data.

the cost of the HIV test was considered an important barrier (see figure 3.8).

Limited availability of HIV testing in public centers and the high cost in countries where coverage is not universal impose barriers to testing and counseling for people infected with HIV/AIDS and people with high-risk behaviors. Overall, these barriers lead to many negative consequences for patients, such as decreased benefits from counseling, early diagnosis, and treatment. Promotion of HIV testing and increased accessibility to the test should be a priority for all Latin American countries.

Figure 3.8. Percentage of NGOs (n = 84) Reporting Barriers to HIV Testing, 2000

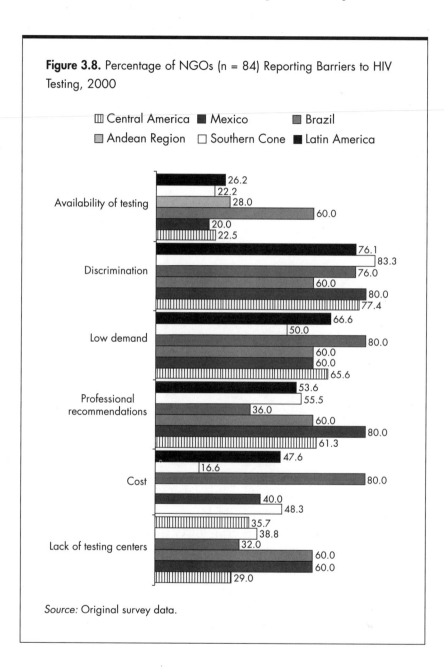

Source: Original survey data.

Table 3.21. Laboratory Testing of CD4 and Viral Load Counts and Cost of HIV/AIDS Health Services, 2000

COUNTRY OR SUBREGION[a]	NUMBER OF LABORATORIES PERFORMING CD4 COUNTS	NUMBER OF CD4 COUNTS PERFORMED	NUMBER OF LABORATORIES TESTING VIRAL LOAD	NUMBER OF VIRAL LOAD TESTS PERFORMED	HIV/AIDS HEALTH SERVICES COSTS (US$)
Mexico	9	920	3	1,831	24,800,000
Central America					
Honduras	2	—	1	—	20,288,461
Nicaragua	1	—	0	—	—
Panama	4	1,200	2	625	—
Brazil	73	207,500	65	203,100	—
Andean Region					
Venezuela, R.B. de	2	12,000	2	12,000	—
Ecuador	0	—	1	—	—
Peru	5	—	3	—	—
Southern Cone					
Argentina	125	—	8	14,760	—
Uruguay	12	2,700	12	1,300	—
Chile	1	5,000	2	6,000	6,116,866

— Not available
a. No data were available from countries not listed.
Source: Original survey data.

Laboratory Infrastructure

According to the national programs, the infrastructure for laboratories working with HIV is underdeveloped. The number of laboratories per country capable of providing CD4 counts[*] is low in Central America, the Andean Region, and Mexico. The number of laboratories that counts viral load[†] is even lower (see table 3.21).

According to the physicians surveyed, in most subregions access to the diagnostic testing needed to evaluate patients and make treatment decisions was limited. Almost half of patients were required to pay for

---

[*]The CD4 count refers to a measure of "helper" T cells, which help B cells produce antibodies. The number of CD4 cells is an important measure of an individual's immune system capacities.
[†]The *Viral load* test is a measure of the amount of HIV in the blood that indicates how far the infection has progressed.

CD4 counts. In general, prices were higher when viral load or resistances were also requested; the highest costs were found in Mexico and Central America (see table 3.22).

According to these physicians, access to basic serologic tests used for clinical evaluation and for antiretroviral treatment planning varied among subregions. Overall, physicians confirmed that about half of HIV-positive patients (48 percent) had had at least one measure of viral load and CD4. Very low coverage was estimated by physicians in Central America and, especially, in Brazil (8 percent and 29 percent respectively; figure 3.9).

Stage of HIV Infection at Time of Diagnosis

Sixty percent of the physicians surveyed stated that patients often did not seek medical attention for the first time until they were already in clinically advanced stages of infection (CDC 1992). In Latin America, 67 percent of HIV-positive people did not seek health care until they were in advanced stages of infection or showed signs and symptoms of AIDS. The longest delays in seeking health services were found in Central America, where eight out of every 10 patients presented with advanced infection or AIDS.

Treatment Coverage

According to the information provided by the physicians surveyed, antiretroviral therapy was provided unequally throughout the region, and there was a significant percentage of PLWHA who lacked the resources to obtain such treatment. In Latin America, one third of HIV-positive patients who should be taking antiretrovirals lacked the resources to do so, while 44 percent of HIV-positive people used highly active antiretroviral therapy (HAART) or multiple combination therapies. Brazil, Mexico, and the Southern Cone provided the greatest coverage of HAART treatment, while low coverage due to lack of resources was more common in Central America, where almost half of HIV-positive patients who should receive antiretroviral therapy (46.5 percent) did not (figure 3.10).

Table 3.22. Percentage of Patients Who Pay for Testing, Cost per Test, and Number of Tests per Patient per Year, 2000

COUNTRY OR SUBREGION	% PATIENTS PAYING FOR CD4 COUNTS	COST PER CD4 COUNT (US$)	CD4 TESTS PER PATIENT PER YEAR	% PATIENTS PAYING FOR VIRAL LOAD COUNTS	COST PER VIRAL LOAD TEST (US$)	VIRAL LOAD COUNT PER PATIENT PER YEAR	% PATIENTS PAYING FOR TESTS OF RESISTANCE	COST PER TEST OF RESISTANCE (US$)	TEST OF RESISTANCE PER PATIENT PER YEAR
Mexico	82.00	83.75	2.20	85.80	125.00	1.60	76.67	491.33	—
Central America (average)	54.56	88.93	2.59	66.47	221.21	2.71	87.50	675.00	1.00
Guatemala	83.33	38.67	1.67	100.00	146.67	1.67	100.00	850.00	—
El Salvador	60.00	113.00	2.40	75.00	265.50	2.20	100.00	—	—
Honduras	67.33	39.33	2.67	100.00	266.67	—	100.00	—	—
Nicaragua	100.00	250.00	2.00	100.00	300.00	3.50	0.00	—	1.00
Costa Rica	0.00	67.50	3.67	0.00	102.50	3.67	0.00	500.00	1.00
Panama	30.00	150.00	4.00	30.00	290.00	4.00	100.00	425.00	
Brazil	0.00	—	3.40	0.00	—	3.20	80.00		
Andean Region (average)	61.59	35.20	2.38	68.00	185.23	2.08	81.82	551.29	0.57
Venezuela, R.B. de	51.25	27.33	2.67	53.75	222.60	2.33	100.00	800.00	0.500
Colombia	26.25	53.25	3.00	50.00	139.50	3.00	50.00	539.75	0.200
Ecuador	70.00	20.00	2.00	52.50	155.00	2.00	100.00	—	
Peru	100.00	30.00	1.33	100.00	246.00	0.67	100.00	450.00	1.00
Bolivia	55.67	20.00	2.50	—	50.00	—	—	—	
Southern Cone (average)	22.27	52.88	3.00	19.82	134.38	2.90	100.00	338.00	2.17
Argentina	11.67	64.33	4.00	5.67	200.00	4.00	100.00	445.00	3.00
Paraguay	10.00	100.00	2.50	10.00	150.00	2.00	—	—	
Uruguay	23.33	0.00	2.00	23.33	0.00	2.00	—		
Chile	40.00	43.33	3.33	37.00	108.33	3.00	100.00	266.67	0.500
Latin America (average)	47.93	63.74	2.67	52.77	181.63	2.52	84.84	485.42	1.275

— Not available.
Source: Original survey data.

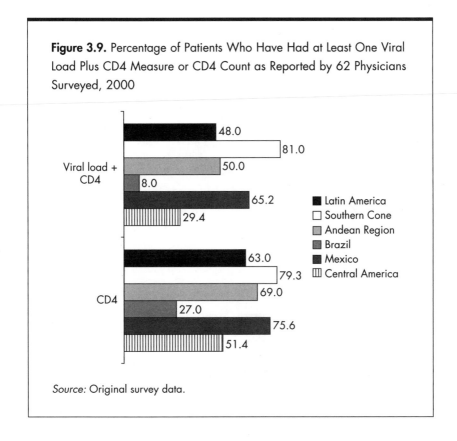

Figure 3.9. Percentage of Patients Who Have Had at Least One Viral Load Plus CD4 Measure or CD4 Count as Reported by 62 Physicians Surveyed, 2000

Source: Original survey data.

According to the national programs, the proportion of patients who needed and received antiretroviral treatment varied. Overall, antiretroviral treatment was provided to half of the patients in Latin America who needed it. Central America and the Andean Region offered the least coverage of antiretroviral treatment (table 3.23).

Prevention of opportunistic infections is another basic component of good clinical practice for treatment of HIV/AIDS. This treatment is inexpensive and is accessible even in areas with few resources. According to the physicians, 72 percent of patients in the region were treated to prevent opportunistic infections. According to those, the countries offering this treatment least were Brazil (13.7 percent), Panama (45 percent), Argentina (55 percent), and Mexico (57 percent).

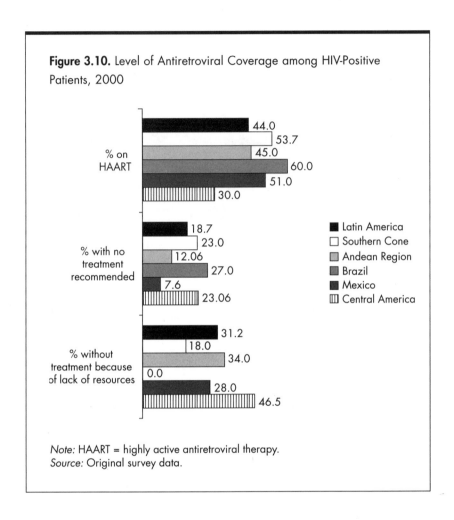

Figure 3.10. Level of Antiretroviral Coverage among HIV-Positive Patients, 2000

Note: HAART = highly active antiretroviral therapy.
Source: Original survey data.

Spending on Antiretrovirals

There was relatively little spending on antiretrovirals in Latin America, which reflects the lack of coverage. According to the national programs, the total spending on antiretroviral therapy in 2000 was US$427 million, including public (US$420.2 million) and private (US$6.7 million) spending. The average cost per patient was estimated at US$7,000 to US$8,000 per patient per year. Considering that there are about 500,000 patients in Latin America who should be treated with antiretrovirals, the spending on this treatment *could* be as high as US$3 billion per year.

Table 3.23. Coverage of Antiretroviral Treatment for Patients Who Need It, According to National Programs, 2000

COUNTRY	PERCENTAGE OF PATIENTS RECEIVING ARV THERAPY
Nicaragua	0
Peru	0
Honduras	<25
Ecuador	<25
Guatemala	25–50
Panama	25–50
Uruguay	50–75
Chile	50–75
Mexico	>75
Costa Rica	>75
Venezuela, R.B. de	>75
Argentina	>75
Paraguay	>75
Brazil	>90
El Salvador	—
Colombia	—
Bolivia	—

— Not available.
Note: ARV = antiretroviral.
Source: Original survey data.

Patient Care

Table 3.24 presents estimates as of 2000 from national programs regarding the proportion of HIV-positive patients who had received health care and psychological or social services during the course of their infection. These estimates include measures such as prophylaxis against opportunistic infections, vaccinations, and antiretroviral treatment. Few people interviewed could provide this information, yet the data available point to some trends that may be indicative of the overall picture. From the information collected, it appears that Central America and the Andean Region were the areas most deficient in terms of services and treatment provided.

To estimate needs for health care and psychological and social services for PLWHA, NGOs were asked to rate on a scale of 1 to 5 the level of concern with certain issues or problems faced by PLWHA,

Table 3.24. Percentage of HIV-Positive Patients Who Have Received Services or Treatments, 2000

COUNTRY[a]	HEALTH CARE	PPD	TB PROPHYLAXIS	PPC PROPHYLAXIS	CMV PROPHYLAXIS	TETANUS VACCINE	PNEUMOCOCO VACCINE	HBV VACCINE	ARV TREATMENT	OPPORTUNISTIC INFECTION TREATMENT	PSYCHOLOGICAL SERVICES	SOCIAL SUPPORT
Mexico	95	30	50	85	2	—	2	10	85	95	40	10
Nicaragua	50	—	—	10	10	20	—	—	—	70	25	30
Venezuela, R.B. de	10	—	—	—	—	—	—	—	10	5	—	—
Paraguay	—	—	100	100	100	100	100	100	100	—	100	100
Uruguay	100	70	100	100	100	—	100	100	100	100	100	100
Chile	100	—	100	100	95	—	100	—	50	60	—	100
Latin America	71	50	83.3	73.8	51.8	60	67.3	55	69	66	66.3	46.7

— Not available.

Note: ARV = antiretroviral; CMV = cytomegalovirus; HBV = hepatitis B virus; PPC = *Pneumocystis carinii* pneumonia; PPD = purified protein derivative, used to test for tuberculosis exposure; TB = tuberculosis.

a. No data were available for countries not listed.

Source: Original survey data.

such as health care, psychological care, employment, social integration, and family and social services. The problems cited as most serious were social discrimination (4.47) and access to employment (4.33). NGOs in Brazil emphasized the problem of discrimination, while in Central America the primary concern was access to employment. Social services for PLWHA are another priority concern in Latin America, particularly in the Southern Cone, Andean Region, and Central America. Concerns regarding psychological and health care services were most frequently cited by NGOs in Mexico and the Andean Region (table 3.25).

Gaps in Health Care Services

Regarding the gaps in health care services, there was a high level of agreement between estimates provided by physicians and national programs surveyed. According to national programs, the primary cause of the most significant health care deficiencies is lack of resources (71 percent), insufficient training for professionals (64 percent), and lack of coordination among the various levels of service providers (64 percent). Responses varied among subregions; for instance, in Central America these three issues were cited in 80 percent of the countries, while in the Andean Region all the countries stated that the main problem was lack of training for professionals. In the Southern Cone the main problems perceived were lack of coordination among various levels and insufficient resources.

Among the physicians surveyed, lack of resources and training were cited as very important problems in the region. Lack of training was considered particularly important in Mexico, Brazil, and the Andean Region. The physicians surveyed attributed gaps in health care services to the following factors: lack of government support or policies (22 percent), low educational level of the population (14 percent), lack of access to antiretrovirals (8 percent), lack of social infrastructure for support (8 percent), and stigmatization of HIV in health care settings (6 percent). Overall, the main finding of this survey is that there are large gaps in health care services provided, and the services offered are very limited.

Table 3.25. Nongovernmental Organizations' Ratings of the Main Problems Faced by PlWHA on a Scale of 1 to 5, 2000

COUNTRY OR SUBREGION	DISCRIMINATION	ACCESS TO EMPLOYMENT	HEALTH SERVICES	SOCIAL SERVICES	PSYCHOLOGICAL SERVICES	FAMILY REJECTION
Mexico	3.50	3.00	4.00	3.75	4.00	2.33
Central America (average)	4.53	4.45	3.81	3.97	3.61	3.47
Guatemala	4.50	4.17	4.67	4.17	3.67	3.50
El Salvador	4.83	4.83	4.67	4.83	4.50	3.33
Honduras	3.75	4.50	2.75	2.50	2.75	2.75
Nicaragua	4.50	4.33	4.67	5.00	3.83	3.67
Costa Rica	5.00	4.80	1.60	2.80	3.20	3.60
Panama	4.50	4.00	3.75	3.75	3.25	4.00
Brazil	4.80	3.80	2.80	2.60	2.60	3.00
Andean Region (average)	4.30	4.18	4.04	4.14	3.48	3.43
Venezuela, R.B. de	4.40	3.80	4.20	3.75	2.00	3.80
Colombia	3.75	5.00	3.25	4.50	4.00	3.50
Ecuador	5.00	3.00	4.00	4.33	3.33	4.00
Peru	3.67	4.00	4.33	4.00	3.33	2.83
Bolivia	5.00	5.00	4.20	4.20	4.20	3.60
Southern Cone (average)	4.72	4.72	3.50	3.94	4.00	3.62
Argentina	5.00	4.60	3.67	3.80	3.50	2.60
Paraguay	5.00	5.00	5.00	5.00	5.00	4.50
Uruguay	4.17	4.83	2.33	3.50	4.20	4.00
Chile	5.00	4.33	3.67	4.00	3.33	3.67
Latin America (average)	4.47	4.33	3.76	3.91	3.61	3.41

Source: Original survey data.

Collaboration with International Agencies

There are many unilateral, bilateral, and multilateral agencies working to control the HIV/AIDS epidemic in Latin American countries. Eighty-five percent of national program respondents estimated that the level of coordination, activities, and prioritization of objectives with these agencies was adequate. With the exception of Colombia, all Latin American countries received funding in 2000 from international agencies. This financing supplemented the funds allocated by governments. The amount of funding received as a proportion of the national HIV/AIDS program budget varied among countries from as low as 1 percent to as high as 40 percent (table 3.26).

Table 3.26. Funding Allocated to National HIV/AIDS Programs from International Agencies and as a Proportion of Governments' HIV/AIDS Budgets, 2000

COUNTRY OR SUBREGION[a]	FUNDING RECEIVED (US$)	PROPORTION OF GOVERNMENT HIV/AIDS BUDGET (%)
Mexico	18,100,000	5.53
Central America		
Guatemala	210,000	3.05
Honduras	1,231,677	0.36
Nicaragua	125,000	0.80
Panama	50,000	—
Brazil	4,500,000	—
Andean Region		
Venezuela, R.B. de	100,000	0.43
Colombia	0.00	0.00
Peru	810,000	6.35
Southern Cone		
Argentina	1,350,000	48.81
Paraguay	37,500	—
Uruguay	110,000	0.72
Latin America (average)	2,420.37	8.26

— Not available.
a. No data were available for countries not listed.
Source: Original survey data.

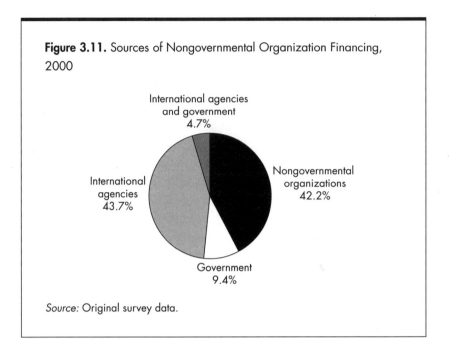

Figure 3.11. Sources of Nongovernmental Organization Financing, 2000

Source: Original survey data.

International Agency Support for NGOs

In Latin America, governments do not provide much funding for NGOs; rather, most of the funding comes from international agencies (43.7 percent) and NGOs' own resources (42.2 percent). Government or ministry of health contributions were scarce, supporting less than 10 percent of programs in the region (figure 3.11).

Principal Barriers and Needs in Controlling the HIV/AIDS Epidemic

National HIV/AIDS Programs

The main problems faced by national HIV/AIDS programs (cited by 45 percent of the respondents from the national programs surveyed) were political indecision on the part of government policy makers and lack of prioritization of the HIV/AIDS epidemic. These problems result in insufficient resource allocation to the fight against

HIV/AIDS (as mentioned by 40 percent of national programs), which further exacerbates the problems these programs face. National program respondents also alluded to the difficulties encountered in reaching high-risk and marginalized populations, problems of under-reporting of HIV and AIDS cases, lack of sufficient training for health care professionals, and the lack of a response and social movement against sexual and social taboos to promote the rights of PLWHA.

Physicians

The group of physicians surveyed associated problems and obstacles mostly with insufficient control and responses from the government, ministry of health, or national program. The issues cited involve policy considerations, technical aspects, and training for professionals. The main barriers mentioned were as follows:

- Inadequate and insufficient information and prevention strategies (62.5 percent)
- Lack of political willingness on the part of governments and national programs (41.7 percent)
- Insufficient epidemiological surveillance (20.8 percent)
- Lack of development of the national program and lack of technical training for national program employees (16.7 percent)
- Religious barriers (16.7 percent)
- Lack of social awareness of the work of NGOs (16.7 percent)
- Discrimination against PLWHA in health care and social settings (12.5 percent)
- Lack of access to antiretrovirals (12.5 percent)
- Lack of sexual education in schools (12.5 percent)
- Lack of access to diagnosis and counseling services (8.3 percent)
- Scarcity of policies for safe blood supplies (4.2 percent).

According to the physicians surveyed, national programs should undertake the following interventions:

- Adequate information and prevention campaigns for the general population as well as high-risk groups (79.0 percent)
- Access to antiretroviral treatment for all HIV-positive patients and for HIV-positive pregnant women (45.2 percent)
- Increased level of political commitment to the fight against HIV/AIDS and increased leadership in national programs (25.0 percent)
- Introduction or expansion of sexual education provided in schools (25.0 percent)
- Improvements to the epidemiological surveillance system for HIV/AIDS (20.8 percent)
- Training for health care personnel and increased sensitivity to HIV/AIDS (12.5 percent)
- Condom promotion (12.5 percent)
- Definition of an adequate legal framework for ensuring the human rights of PLWHA (12.5 percent)
- Increased resources for diagnostic services (8.3 percent)
- Blood safety programs (8.3 percent)
- Programs for IDUs (4.2 percent)
- Consensus on guidelines for diagnosis and treatment of HIV/AIDS (4.2 percent)
- Incorporation of clinical perspectives in decisions made by national programs (4.2 percent).

Nongovernmental Organizations

The group of Latin American NGOs included in the study attributed problems in controlling the epidemic to three primary factors:

(1) government policies (or lack thereof), (2) unmet needs in national programs' activities, and (3) cultural and social values.

Sixty-four percent of all the NGOs surveyed, and 70 percent of NGOs in the Southern Cone, felt that governments were to blame for political indecision, lack of resources for HIV/AIDS programs, limited access to health services, inadequate legislation, and lack of policies for early sexual education. National HIV/AIDS plans, in particular, were strongly criticized from technical perspectives; 78 percent of NGOs[6] made reference to the following aspects:

- Limited capacity to obtain and disseminate high-quality information about the dimensions of the epidemic
- Lack of a structured, multisectorial plan for responding to the epidemic
- Lack of training for technicians responsible for controlling the epidemic at both the national and local levels
- Lack of resources for prevention activities and inadequate or ineffective interventions
- Lack of sensitivity to the need for sexual education
- High cost and lack of access to HIV testing.

According to 46 percent of the NGOs surveyed, the community was also responsible for certain problems in fighting HIV/AIDS, such as:

- Cultural and social barriers to sexual dialogue and education
- Macho attitudes that foster discrimination against women and homophobia
- Poverty and low sociocultural and socioeconomic standing
- Stigmatization of PLWHA.

Sixteen percent of NGOs felt that the Catholic Church blocked many prevention activities, and 10 percent mentioned lack of health coverage and access to antiretrovirals as key problems.

The NGOs surveyed proposed the following interventions to improve efforts to control the HIV/AIDS epidemic:

- *Governments:* Stronger policy decisions, including prioritization of policies regarding HIV/AIDS and sexual education in schools; increased resources; promotion of citizens' movements; and strict penalties for violations of human rights and discrimination against PLWHA (mentioned by 43 percent of all NGOs and 62 percent of Central American NGOs)

- *National programs:* Training for employees and technicians of national programs; prevention campaigns for high-risk groups; incorporation of sexual education in schools; development of multisectorial strategies with the capacity to coordinate the work among different sectors; dissemination of more accurate information about the epidemic; and introduction and expansion of policies for integrated, comprehensive management of patients with HIV/AIDS (mentioned by 94 percent of NGOS)

- *Communities:* Promote human rights and equality, especially sexual equality (mentioned by 7 percent of all NGOs and 12 percent of Central American NGOs)

- *Health sectors:* Improve access to health services and antiretroviral treatments (mentioned by 9 percent of all NGOs and 18 percent of NGOs in Central America).

The NGOs surveyed were also asked to identify barriers to implementing the above-mentioned interventions. Ninety-one percent of NGOs in Central America and Mexico, as well as 85 percent of NGO groups in the Southern Cone, mentioned lack of government policy support. National programs were considered to be responsible for lack of coordination and resources for NGOs and lack of attention and services for high-risk groups by 56 percent of Central American and Mexican NGOs and 61 percent of Southern Cone NGOs. Thirty-five percent of Central American NGOs surveyed felt that the Catholic Church would be a barrier due to the lack of separation of church and state, while 30 percent of NGOs in the Andean Region,

Brazil, and the Southern Cone felt that the community itself would be a barrier in terms of the prevailing macho attitudes and other cultural stereotypes.

Notes

1. Peru and Bolivia are not included; no data were available.

2. Here, *program* refers to an organized, systematized, and coherent group of integrated activities and services that are carried out with allocated resources and a goal of reaching previously determined objectives related to preventing new HIV infections in a defined population. This term does not refer to occasional activities, one-time activities, or activities that respond to an immediate, urgent demand.

3. Respondents from four countries provided data on needle exchange programs and units. In 2000, Uruguay had no needle exchange programs, Mexico had one program and one unit, Argentina had five programs (no data were provided on units), and Brazil had 125 programs and 125 units.

4. *CD4 count* refers to a measure of helper T cells that help B cells produce antibodies. The number of CD4 cells is an important measure of an individual's immune system capacities.

5. *Viral load test* is a measure of the amount of HIV in the blood to determine how far infection has progressed.

6. Central American NGOs were even more critical of national programs, with 85 percent citing these problems.

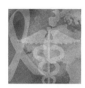

CHAPTER 4

Key Areas for Interventions and Challenges Ahead

Summary

Despite relatively high rates of HIV infection in most countries and the lack of effective interventions carried out thus far, Latin America has the necessary infrastructure to efficiently and effectively confront the HIV/AIDS epidemic, if provided with the necessary resources. This chapter highlights the main areas in need of improvement, strategies that might make national responses more effective, and the principal challenges to implementation.

High-risk groups constitute the majority of HIV infection and are the groups most likely to spread HIV, yet interventions for these groups are still not widespread. The implementation of interventions for these groups, as well as school-based sexual education and HIV/AIDS information programs, stands to contribute greatly to the fight against HIV/AIDS. Effective guidelines for prevention interventions are needed. Review and revision of blood safety policies would begin the process of achieving universal testing of donated blood and acceptance of only voluntary, altruistic, nonremunerated blood donations. Multisectorial coordination is an indispensable condition for producing synergies and long-lasting social and political agreement and for increasing the intensity and scope of interventions.

Health care coverage and social and psychological support are also key challenges. Health care coverage is a necessary condition for improving impacts and guaranteeing the effectiveness of interventions, yet many people infected with HIV do not have access to health care. Lack of resources and medical training are the main deficiencies within the health care setting. Promotion of HIV testing, especially among high-risk populations, is a basic and essential strategy, and expansion of centers for anonymous diagnosis, counseling, and treatment is urgently needed for early diagnosis, health care access, treatment, and prevention. The coverage of current interventions for decreasing mother-to-child transmission of HIV requires more action, since coverage is still low. Universal availability of HIV testing to pregnant women and incorporation of HIV testing into the battery of prenatal diagnostic tests would help prevent mother-to-child transmission. At the same time, social and psychological support services are still poor and limited.

By including a fight against ignorance and promotion of human rights in the messages delivered to the general population, health and social services personnel would help ensure the right to health care, "normalization" of HIV/AIDS, access to HIV testing, and implementation of universal precautions. Indeed, these factors are the key elements for reducing rejection based on bias and social stigma and increasing knowledge.

There is a need for more information about the epidemic and its trends. One of the main priorities is the production of high-quality epidemiological information for decision making. To this end, technicians working for national programs need training in prevention, management, and epidemiological surveillance.

Based on the findings of this study, the main challenges to meeting the current needs are availability of resources; institutional capacity to provide training in all areas; and cultural, social, and religious factors. Coordinated and targeted interventions from various agencies, NGOs, and governments may guide future regionwide interventions.

Introduction

As in many countries, the multiplicity of health problems affecting Latin America inhibited recognition of the need for a dedicated, tailored response to the HIV/AIDS epidemic and of its serious consequences in terms of morbidity and mortality and its capacity for aggravating existing health problems (e.g., TB and other infectious diseases). As a result, HIV/AIDS was not given priority among health concerns until international organizations and social movements gained significant social and political importance and the epidemic demonstrated how lethal it could be, not only in terms of health care, but also in terms of social and economic consequences.

Since the late 1980s Latin American countries have confronted the HIV/AIDS epidemic by creating new structures and showing the social fabric necessary to promote community responses (Bolivia 2000b; Colombia 2000; Honduras 1999; Nicaragua 2000; Guatemala 1999, 2000; Costa Rica 2001; Peru 2001). Latin American national HIV/AIDS programs have a tradition of carving out their own unique roles and responsibilities within ministries of health and have benefited from the involvement of multidisciplinary professionals and sectors.

There has been tremendous progress in management capacity and articulating social responses. Latin America has an excellent framework for effective interventions with multilateral and bilateral organizations; the resources, infrastructure, and professionals are in place to implement a variety of interventions, evaluate their impact, and sustain them over time. However, the capacity to respond has been limited by political, technical, and social problems. These limitations were confirmed by the national program directors, health professionals, and NGOs interviewed for our survey.

Despite the political commitment of governments to confront the epidemic, as evidenced by the prioritization of HIV/AIDS in health care agendas and the HIV/AIDS-related legislation throughout the region, limited resources and high turnover of personnel have been serious obstacles to fully effective responses. The technical capacity of national entities to offer a stronger response has been constrained by the same problems. A significant proportion of physicians mentioned deficiencies in prevention strategies (62 percent), epidemiological surveillance (20 percent), and technical capacity of professionals working in national programs (16 percent). NGOs were even more concerned with the technical training needs for national program professionals; 78 percent mentioned this problem. Finally, social, cultural, and religious values have also been significant barriers to an adequate response to the epidemic in certain subregions.

Overall, the survey results show a high level of consensus among physicians and NGOs, shared to a lesser degree by national programs, regarding the problems faced in fighting HIV/AIDS.

This chapter synthesizes the areas in need of improvement and recommends strategies that may make national responses more effective, taking into account the principal challenges to implementation. As a whole, this document also aims to help countries tailor the Global Strategy Framework (Joint United Nations Programme on HIV/AIDS [UNAIDS] 2001b) to their local context, depending on the key problems identified.

These recommendations are intended to strengthen the health sector response in terms of expanding its influence in neglected areas and entering into multisectorial partnerships. Finally, although this chapter does not delve into the roles and responsibilities of other sectors, it takes into account the advances in strategic thinking and the elements of a successful multisectorial response to the epidemic.

National Response to the Epidemic: Prevention

Key Problems

Although there have been numerous programs and campaigns for the general population, fewer prevention activities for high-risk groups have been conducted in many countries. The reason for this could be a substantial lack of information on the level of infection and trends in these groups. With the exception of Mexico and Honduras, the respondents from national programs felt that they did not have the data they needed on prevalence rates in different populations and that data were inconsistent when different sources were compared.

Information collected from respondents showed that men who have sex with men (MSM) have been the target of prevention programs in most countries, although there were gaps in some Central American and Southern Cone countries. At the same time, according to those interviewed, 41 percent of countries developed programs for commercial sex workers (CSWs) as late as 1999–2000, and they were not widespread in all subregions.

In the most affected areas, interventions for injecting drug users (IDUs) were still insufficient. Harm reduction programs were relatively new in Argentina, Chile, Mexico, and Brazil, and their scope depended on the level of political commitment; a favorable legal framework; and the capacity for health, social, and community responses to the problem of injecting drug use. Recent adoption of new policies has led to interventions that meet the needs in these countries, but at the same time, respondents from countries strongly affected, such as Colombia and Paraguay, did not claim to have programs, and data collected from Uruguay showed only drug-free programs, which are not as effective as harm reduction programs.

Although 70 percent of countries stated that they had programs for prisoners, with the exception of Mexico respondents reported that these programs were only recently started (1999–2000) and that coverage was low. Honduras and most countries from the Andean Region lacked programs for prisoners. Aside from the challenges of expanding health education programs and counseling and promoting diagnostic testing and condom use, there is the additional challenge of introducing harm reduction programs and coordinating with external health services, especially in prisons with high rates of injecting drug use.

Health and sexual education programs for adolescents and young people are the most widespread interventions in Latin America. According to the respondents, 47 percent of countries had school-based programs, and 29 percent carried out occasional activities, yet the contents were not always appropriate because of religious or cultural censorship, social conservatism, and frequent political veto. Of those interviewed, 25 percent of physicians and 90 percent of NGOs mentioned the need to improve and expand these programs. In terms of high-risk groups, respondents from only half the countries surveyed indicated that they had programs for adolescents who did not go to school or those considered to be at high risk. The promotion of condom use by young people has met cultural and religious barriers, which are significant challenges to the control of the HIV/AIDS epidemic.

Interventions for the general population, which were reported as more widespread and frequent in the region, have not always obtained the anticipated results in creating the climate of solidarity and confidence necessary for effective prevention, according to the perception of the respondents. Study data indicated that the frequency of campaigns in the last 10 years was low in the Southern Cone and Andean Region. Only 25 percent of countries had programs for promoting condom use, despite the fact that sexual transmission is the most prevalent transmission mode in Latin America. Seventy-nine percent of physicians felt that it was necessary to develop better prevention strategies for the general population and high-risk groups. Indeed, there is a significant difference between the more widespread interventions for the general population, with greater visibility and political impact, and those for high-risk groups, which are much more cost-effective mechanisms for controlling the spread of the epidemic.

In terms of multisectoriality, Latin American countries have developed strategic plans with participation by a broad range of stakeholders (e.g., government ministries, civil society, associations of PLWHA, bilateral and multilateral partners), and they serve as the common reference for action. Now, plans are ready to become reality. Data from the survey respondents show that the levels of multisectorial coordination were unequal among countries in the region. The study also showed that although there were structures in place to foster multisectorial coordination in almost all countries, the level of true collaboration was still low due to a lack of resources and coverage for coordinated execution of interventions.

Community-based movements have a strong tradition in Latin America, primarily in countries with more economic potential and where there are government-financed programs (e.g., Southern Cone countries, Brazil, and Mexico). However, most Latin American NGOs finance their own programs or receive financing from international agencies; only 34 percent of NGOs surveyed had received government funding in the last five years. The level of NGO representation in national programs and commissions was high, and 67 percent of the NGOs surveyed belonged to national committees. Still, NGO respondents indicated that there was limited coordination between NGOs and governments in interventions for specific populations.

NGOs are much more likely to have access to marginal populations or those that lack health services, yet most NGOs and governments have dedicated the majority of their efforts to groups with "variable risk" for infection (e.g., the general population, young people, women). Almost half of the targeted NGO programs (48 percent) were focused on young people and women, while CSWs or MSM were the focus of only 25 percent of such programs.

Interventions Addressing the Problems Identified

Social Mobilization and Community Responses

Approaches that focus on social mobilization and building community responses should combine and reinforce strategies for risk, vulnerability, and impact reduction. Stronger involvement and continued pressure from civil society may be the only way to expand the response to HIV/AIDS in the near future. It is essential to strengthen civil society organizations dealing with HIV/AIDS as well as those working on development, human rights, gender, and other issues. Ultimately, communities and civil society, including associations of PLWHA, are the basis of the response to HIV/AIDS in the region.

High-Risk Groups

Interventions for high-risk groups should be intensified, since this is where the highest levels of infection are found, and since they are the groups most likely to spread HIV to other groups and the general population (World Bank 1997). The interventions could combine risk reduction with other strategies that focus on vulnerability and impact reduction, which implies decreased stigma, policy development, and care and support that work to create incentives for early detection, thereby reinforcing prevention efforts.

Multisectorial Coordination

Multisectorial coordination, in government and NGOs, is an indispensable condition for producing partnerships, fomenting long-lasting social and political agreement, and increasing the intensity and scope of interventions.

Sexual Transmission

In all Latin American countries, sexual activity is the most prevalent way HIV is spread, which means that it is critical to have interventions focused on decreasing the risk of infection for MSM, CSWs, and people with sexually transmitted infections (STIs) and multiple partners. Strategies that have proved their effectiveness include counseling, health education, condom use promotion, promotion of HIV testing, management of STIs, and promotion and preservation of human rights (National Institutes of Health 2000; Cohen and Eron 2001; Rotheram-Borus, Cantwell, and Newman 2000; Merson, Dayton, and O'Reilly 2000; CDC 1999a; Weinhardt and others 1999; UNAIDS 2000g, 2001c; Kelly 2000; Fleming and Wasserheit 1999). Collaboration with STI clinics, creation of a network of anonymous diagnosis centers, and access to free services are key elements for successful programs.

Collaboration with gay organizations in planning programs for MSM would do much for the development of services and prevention messages that respond to the needs and communication norms of this group (Kegeles and others 1999). The network of MSM for Latin America and the Caribbean could strengthen effective approaches focused on promoting social mobilization and building community responses.

Due to their constant exposure to risk, male and female CSWs are a key group in prevention of HIV/AIDS (World Bank 2001; UNAIDS 2000l; Ghys, Jenkins, and Pisani 2001; Scalway 2001). Interventions to decrease vulnerability for CSWs are highly cost-effective in terms of reducing the possibility of transmitting HIV to clients (usually men) and their partners (often women of childbearing age and possibly their children) (Piot and Coll 2001). A variable percentage of CSWs are also injecting drug users, so their risk of becoming infected is even greater. Therefore, harm reduction programs (needle exchange or distribution of kits or sterile needles) might do well by targeting areas frequented by CSWs, especially in countries where IDU prevalence rates are high. Male CSWs are exposed to even greater risk, given the frequency of services they provide to other men (Belza and others 2001). Finally, transvestite and transsexual CSWs require specially tailored programs because of their unique sociocultural characteristics and sexual identity.

Access to health centers and STI clinics for CSWs plays an important role in preventing transmission, promoting HIV testing, and diagnosing and treating STIs (Ghys and others 2001; Levine and others 1998). Ideally, these centers would offer free services and be accessible to all CSWs, men and women, regardless of where they work.

Injecting Drug Use

IDUs are one of the groups most at risk for contracting HIV and disseminating it to the general population. A substantial proportion of IDUs rarely use health services, so it is important to implement community-based outreach programs (Hughes 1977; Stimson and others 1994). With the exception of Brazil and Mexico, such programs have been scarcely developed in Latin America. Harm reduction programs are most effective for preventing transmission of HIV and other blood-borne diseases, as well as for achieving higher quality of life and health for IDUs (Des Jarlais and others 1995). In the most affected countries, there is a need for the initiation or expansion of harm reduction programs that address the specific substances injected (e.g., heroin, cocaine). Programs for needle exchange, training on how to clean injecting drug equipment, outreach programs for drug addicts, and diagnosis of HIV and other infections are crucial for treating this high-risk group (UNAIDS 2001a; United Nations 2000; Hartgers and others 1989; Kaplan, Khoshnood, and Heimer 1994; van Ameijden and others 1995; Laufer 2001; Wood and others 2001). Prevention of sexual transmission is another challenge for IDUs, since they place their partners at great risk of becoming infected. Mass condom distribution associated with harm reduction programs and health education for IDUs and their friends, families, and partners are much-needed interventions. Given the needs for prevention, health care, and social resources, mobile units for dissemination of prevention materials and needle exchange are potentially key resources for guaranteeing the coverage and continuity of interventions.

Young People

Intensifying programs for reducing vulnerability with a focus on adolescents and young people is an essential step. To this end, sexual education and HIV/AIDS information for adolescents and young people are key (ONUSIDA 1997b). Integration of such programs into school curriculums and involvement of ministries of education in these activities would guarantee continuity and expansion of school-based HIV/AIDS and sexual education and peer relations that model safer behaviors. These programs would reinforce condom use, making condoms accessible to young people through distribution in areas frequented by young people in schools and universities (ONUSIDA 1997b). There is also a significant percentage of children who do not go to school (especially in Central America). In such cases, it is necessary to implement health and sexual education activities outside of the school environment. Outreach programs can be very effective for reaching these children.

Prisoners

Due to the high-risk environment in which they live, prisoners also require interventions (ONUSIDA 1997a). Health education and human rights programs are fundamental for creating favorable conditions for behavior change for prisoners. Active participation of prison health authorities and responsible ministries is crucial for the expansion and continuity of these activities. Promotion of voluntary HIV testing, access to health care (Sabin and others 2001), diagnosis and treatment of STIs, condom distribution, and harm reduction programs for IDUs (Nelles and others 1998) are important elements in the control of HIV in prisons (Inciardi 1996). These services could be coordinated with health and preventive services working with the general population (Rich and others 2001) since many prisoners will eventually be released and will require further treatment, particularly prisoners who are also IDUs.

Women and Girls

The HIV/AIDS impact on women and girls calls for strong efforts addressing the factors that place them in disadvantaged situations, increasing their risk (e.g., inability to negotiate sex, lack of access to preventive services) and decreasing their sense of control over their own lives. Gender policies that strengthen and build women's empowerment and capacity for sexual negotiation are very effective (ONUSIDA 2000b), especially for women at high risk (e.g., sexual partners of IDUs or PLWHA, women with STIs, residence in high prevalence areas), but are underdeveloped in Latin America.

Analysis of this situation justifies the development of policies and interventions to reduce vulnerability at the individual and community levels and demonstrates a need for continuous coordination between governments and NGOs, including an increase in the participation of NGOs in planning national responses to the epidemic. Indeed, coordination among governments, NGOs, and international financing agencies is an urgent need given the lack of strategies that could help reduce the risk of infection and its negative consequences in high-risk populations, especially those most marginalized (CSWs,

IDUs, and MSM in certain sectors of the population) and most reachable through NGO-led interventions.

Access to Health and Social Services

Key Problems

It is estimated that a substantial proportion of people infected with HIV do not have adequate health care. The reasons for this are diverse, including limited access to services, the cost of services (including those provided in public hospitals), clinical care below quality standards, lack of infrastructure for prevention programs in health care environments, and insufficient psychological and social services. Only six countries in Latin America offer universal health care coverage (Costa Rica, Brazil, the República Bolivariana de Venezuela, Argentina, Chile, and Paraguay); in the other countries, health care is guaranteed for clients with insurance, while the rest must pay out of pocket for services. In Central America, coverage under social security systems is scarce, and payment for services is more common. The cost of HIV testing is high, even in public centers; the average cost of the test is US$20.

In Latin America, there are few clinical management guidelines for HIV/AIDS that are reasonable in relation to countries' resources, particularly in the Southern Cone and the Andean Region, and guidelines for prophylaxis indications were reported in only 15.6 percent of countries in the region.

Physicians and national program representatives surveyed in this study agreed that medical training is one of the main deficiencies in health care. This was mentioned as an important problem by government officials (especially in Central America) and physicians throughout the countries surveyed. Respondents from Mexico, Brazil, and the Andean Region considered their countries most in need of improvement.

All three groups surveyed (physicians, NGOs, and national programs) provided inconsistent information regarding the availability of prevention programs in health centers; only national programs confirmed the availability of such programs. Psychological and social services were considered insufficient by governments, physicians, and NGOs.

According to the physicians surveyed, 63 percent of patients received adequate clinical management, according to current quality standards. Central American countries (primarily Honduras and Nicaragua) and the Andean Region were working to improve the quality of clinical care provided. In the physicians' opinion, coverage of prophylactic measures against opportunistic infections was estimated at only 13 percent in Brazil and from 45 percent to 57 percent in Panama, Argentina, and Mexico; regional coverage was about 72 percent.

New antiretroviral therapies have resulted in increased quality of life and survival for PLWHA (Hammer and others 1997; Palella and others 1998). However, the situation is not so simple—treatment must be followed for a lifetime; insufficient prescriptions, misuse, or missed doses can generate resistances and increase the possibility of transmitting resistant strains of the virus (Carpenter and others 1998). For antiretroviral therapy to be effective, broad health resources infrastructure is needed, including specialized laboratories and infectious disease services in hospitals capable of complying with quality standards. By strengthening current infrastructure and training physicians, the region could soon use new treatments more effectively. According to estimates from the surveyed physicians and governments, between 44 percent and 55 percent of PLWHA receive antiretroviral therapy, yet there is wide disparity among countries; coverage is notably low in Central America.

Health resources infrastructure varies in terms of levels of development and accessibility throughout Latin America. Many countries are immersed in reform processes, which can affect the level of attention given to patients and the quality of health care. At the same time, there are general deficiencies in areas such as resources infrastructure, especially the network of HIV diagnostic laboratories and labs for determining CD4 levels and viral load, as well as infrastructure for diagnosis and follow-up on coinciding infections and other disease processes associated with HIV/AIDS. According to the national programs, the network of laboratories is insufficient, especially in Central America and the Andean Region. Access to services is limited by the payment required; almost half of patients must pay out of pocket for CD4 level tests, and even more must pay for viral load testing. Consequently, only half of PLWHA (48 percent) had had at least one viral load and CD4 test, according to the physicians surveyed. Coverage in Brazil and Central America was particularly low, at 8 percent and 29 percent respectively.

There is an unquantified, yet substantial, proportion of infected people who do not know that they are HIV positive and who will probably know only when late, undeniable symptoms of infection are present. According to the physicians surveyed, 67 percent of people infected with HIV/AIDS seek access to services for the first time at advanced stages of infection or when they have already progressed to AIDS. The latest diagnoses are found in Central America, where eight out of every 10 patients first seek access to health services with advanced infection or AIDS. This situation is even more serious for women planning to have children or pregnant women, because in these cases early diagnosis is essential to ensure access to treatments that may prevent mother-to-child transmission. Overall, improvements are needed for early diagnosis, access to counseling, and follow-up lab testing. Although more than 50 percent of physicians and NGOs participating in the study felt that HIV testing was accessible, there were still barriers to coverage that have implications for supply and demand. These barriers include discrimination, specificity or uniqueness of the test and consequently the unlikelihood of it being offered in most clinics, cost, availability of health centers, and the test itself.

Finally, interventions for decreasing mother-to-child transmission of HIV in health centers require more action, since coverage is still low, according to the survey. Only 52 percent of pregnant women in Latin America were offered the HIV test; Central America and Mexico had the lowest rates of offering HIV testing to pregnant women. Even more worrisome is the fact that only 56 percent of HIV-positive pregnant women received antiretroviral prophylaxis, which can prevent mother-to-child transmission.

Interventions for Addressing the Problems Identified

All interventions aimed at improving health and social services require multisectorial collaboration (UNAIDS 2000v). Coordination among those responsible for health and social services in governments, regions, states, and municipalities is key.

In many countries, it is necessary to expand coverage of health services for HIV/AIDS patients in order to provide maximum quality of care (clinical follow-up, prophylaxis against opportunistic infections, diagnosis and treatment of pathology associated with HIV/AIDS, and palliative care for terminally ill patients). There are certain prerequisites that could make this possible, including strengthening the network of health centers and hospitals; increasing services for people without health care coverage; and training physicians, pediatricians, and nurses in clinical management and treatment of HIV and other STIs. In addition, expansion and wide coverage of quality health care for HIV/AIDS is one of the key elements for guaranteeing the effectiveness of antiretroviral therapy (Pan American Health Organization [PAHO] 2000a).

Promotion of HIV testing, especially among high-risk populations, is a basic strategy at the regional level. Expansion of centers for anonymous diagnosis, counseling, and treatment would help reach the goal of adequate coverage, early diagnosis, and health care for PLWHA, as well as prevention for those who are at high risk (CDC 2001a; Summers and others 2000). When such services are well publicized in different communities, problems of discrimination and stigmatization are avoided, and populations who would not get the test elsewhere are attracted. Health care professionals in these centers require training in prevention, education, counseling, and management of emotionally difficult situations. Training in syndromic management of STIs is also highly recommended.

Universal offering of HIV testing to pregnant women and its incorporation into the battery of prenatal diagnostic tests would go a long way toward preventing mother-to-child transmission (UNAIDS 1999a, 1999b; CDC 2001b; International Perinatal HIV Group 1999). The current guidelines for clinical management, treatment for pregnant women, and prophylaxis with antiretroviral therapy may be followed only when services are adequately and appropriately planned, so collaboration with professional associations of gynecology, obstetrics, midwifery, community health workers, pediatrics, managers of prenatal services, and citizens organizations is imperative. Taking this a step further, maternal and child postpartum care is also important, including counseling on continued care needed and feeding strategies.

Laboratory networks are in need of strengthening and expansion in all of Latin America in order to ensure that services offered meet the needs of patients. Laboratories conducting CD4 and viral load tests may work toward carrying out at least two tests per year per patient. Training for laboratory technicians is also necessary to ensure knowledge of current and upcoming techniques, as well as of tests used for diagnosis and determining resistances.

Policies for multisectorial integration also have implications for physicians, whose representation and voice in national programs has been lacking. Partnerships and dialogue between physicians and national programs would help to develop guidelines and recommendations for clinical management and treatment based on current quality standards and adapted to the patients' needs and resources available. Such collaboration would also guarantee consideration of the physicians' perspective when decisions are made by national programs.

Human Rights

Key Problems

Among the main barriers to improved effectiveness of programs and expanding access to prevention and clinical care are lack of information, stigmatization, homophobia, and social prejudices regarding sexual orientation or behavior. These barriers affect the general population, as well as health care and social services professionals. Ninety-four percent of the NGOs surveyed confirmed social or legal restrictions on homosexuality. There are still significant barriers preventing PLWHA from accessing health centers, which impedes fair and equitable treatment and generates more stigmatization and rejection. Interventions to address these issues are scarce, and there are numerous obstacles that people at high risk or that are HIV-positive face when trying to access services for prevention, diagnosis, and treatment. In terms of human rights for PLWHA, discrimination and employment difficulties (primarily regarding access) were the main challenges mentioned by Latin American NGOs.

Interventions That Address the Problems Identified

A fight against ignorance and promotion of human rights should be part of the message delivered to the general population as well as to health and social services personnel (Busza 2001). Communication and media messages about the right to health care (De Cock and Johnson 1998), "normalization" of HIV/AIDS, access to HIV testing, and implementation of universal precautions would help to reduce rejection and stigmatization of PLWHA in the health care environment.

In coordination with national education authorities and interdisciplinary teams, programs addressing the issue of schooling for HIV-positive children would benefit many through guaranteeing the right to an education.

The right to work and integration or reintegration into the workforce (CDC 1987a, 1988, 1989) should be reinforced through a collaborative effort with ministries of labor and social issues; this is crucial for reducing stigmatization of HIV/AIDS. In addition, equal work conditions for PLWHA are fair and just measures, as is voluntary access to health checkups and transparency of health screening in order to avoid possible discrimination and other negative consequences faced by PLWHA.

Involving PLWHA in all strategies for prevention and control of the epidemic is a key to success. This involvement can work to reduce stigma and discrimination toward PLWHA and radically change their position in society.

Finally, the right to access health, social, and psychological services and to a dignified death must be ensured and is particularly a challenge for NGOs, justice authorities, and prison institutions.

National Capacity: Structure and Management

Key Problems

All countries have multisectorial plans to confront the epidemic, but the actual functionality and capacity for a collaborative response have been mediated by the technical and political capacity of national programs and by the limited resources available for HIV/AIDS control. Forty-one percent of physicians surveyed identified the need to strengthen leadership in national programs and create greater political commitment, while 94 percent of NGOs mentioned the need to strengthen training and improve interventions in national programs. The level of integration and commitment of community-based movements and the creation of networks are still limited in most countries. Thus, most social and psychological services for PLWHA are provided by NGOs; government involvement is lacking. International agencies have an important role in responding to the epidemic and financing national programs and many Latin American NGOs. Although most national programs stated that the level of coordination with international agencies was high, the programs implemented through such collaborative efforts did not always meet the needs of the population. For instance, 48 percent of NGO programs targeted populations that were easy to access through multisectorial structures or programs, which neglects high-risk and hard-to-reach populations.

Health sector reforms currently under way are another obstacle to plans for integrated HIV/AIDS services in Latin America, but eventually advancement of these reforms will result in greater coordination among different levels of specialization and complexity and progressive incorporation of prevention strategies into the services provided. In clinical management of HIV/AIDS patients, prevention is an essential component that may benefit not only the patient, but also his or her friends, family, and partners (MacNeil and Anderson 1998; Ruiz and others 2000).

Epidemiological surveillance systems in Latin America vary in terms of level of development, but their overall capacity to provide the information needed is low. Availability of systematized information on the incidence of newly diagnosed HIV infections and sentinel surveillance coverage (especially among the most affected groups) is scarce throughout the region. Registries of AIDS cases, which have existed the longest, suffer high levels of underreporting in certain subregions, especially Central America. Consequently, services and programs are planned, interventions are evaluated, and decisions are made based on partial information that is not always adequate for decision making. Surveillance infrastructure is limited, and there is a critical need for technical training for surveillance professionals to attain greater quality and applicability of information generated, particularly in Central America. Higher levels of development and implementation are needed in the surveillance of HIV infection, behavioral risk factors, and the information systems used to better meet the current needs. The main challenge for epidemiological surveillance is to develop activities based on the characteristics and evolution of the epidemic, with an aim toward sustainability over time and capacity to produce data that are comparable and consistent at the national and international levels.

The safety of blood supply programs is heterogeneous throughout the region, so blood and blood products are not as safe as desired in certain countries. Indeed, in most countries less than 100 percent of donated blood is screened for HIV. The greatest deficiencies in blood testing were found in Central America and the Andean Region, particularly Bolivia, where increased coverage is urgently needed. Blood donation policies have not been adapted to meet the necessary quality standards in which donation is exclusively voluntary, altruistic, and nonremunerated. For instance, aside from Argentina, Brazil, and Honduras, where blood donation is always voluntary and never remunerated, the rest of the Latin American countries also allow remunerated donations, which have been proved to be less safe.

Interventions That Address the Problems Identified

Ministries of health and national programs require improved and increased infrastructure and resources to consolidate and lead multisectorial national responses to the HIV/AIDS epidemic. Active participation of NGOs, states, regions, municipalities, and international agencies is imperative for establishing prevention and control policies, especially for high-risk and vulnerable populations. To this end, NGO networks deserve much encouragement and support. Such networks would coordinate interventions and, with national programs, prioritize the main areas for activities.

One of the main priorities is the production of adequate and appropriate epidemiological information for decision making (UNAIDS 2000n; Schwartlander and others 2001; McFarland and Cáceres 2001; Des Jarlais, Dehne, and Casabona 2001). Training programs covering methodology, epidemiological surveillance, and data for decision making are needed for all those working in surveillance. National plans for epidemiological surveillance containing priorities and specific working protocols are urgently needed for homogenizing and increasing efficiency in the production of information. The involvement of physicians and public and private health centers is fundamental for reducing underreporting.

Guidelines for prevention interventions are needed that consolidate those interventions that have been most effective. These guidelines would have the consensus of the different actors involved and would include protocols for programs targeting different groups. Interventions are needed at different levels in order to reach those at greatest risk. The elimination or minimization of legal barriers to prevention methods and health care for IDUs (e.g., legalized sale and distribution of sterile needles), MSM (elimination of discriminatory norms), and CSWs (ensured access to health care) would greatly improve efforts in these high-risk groups.

Ideally, blood safety policies would be revised to achieve universal testing of donated blood and acceptance of only voluntary, altruistic, nonremunerated donations.

In order to cover all these needs and improvements, it is necessary to guarantee that personnel are trained in epidemiological surveillance, HIV/AIDS prevention, coordination with NGOs and other government or regional institutions, planning, blood and blood products control and safety, clinical management, and management of health care services. To guarantee the efficacy and sustainability of the interventions needed, the continuity of professionals, in terms of roles and positions, must be ensured within the scope of HIV/AIDS services.

Main Challenges in Implementing the Recommended Interventions

The difficulties in carrying out a more effective response to the HIV/AIDS epidemic are multiple and, in many cases, similar to those facing the responses to other health problems in Latin America.

An increase in available resources is a key element for confronting the epidemic. In the last five years, multilateral organizations such as UNAIDS have stimulated the creation of networks for linking national programs to analyze and design responses throughout the region. However, policy strength and international involvement have not always led to increased budgets or greater political willingness to create solid, sustainable organizations and structures.

Another substantial problem lies in the institutional capacity to provide a response that is effective and the capacity of universities to ensure that the response is within the range of professional training (e.g., clinical, prevention, epidemiological surveillance, planning). The continuity of professionals with appropriate technical training is subject to political changes, availability of sufficient personnel, and resources, which are handicaps for the consistency and quality of interventions implemented.

Finally, cultural, social, and religious factors constitute barriers that, in many countries, obstruct good technical proposals or government decisions that could protect the public health and the overall well-being of citizens. In virtually all of Latin America, it is very difficult to separate religious and cultural beliefs from the role of the state.

Conclusions

Strategies for addressing HIV/AIDS are tailored to different settings based on the unique dynamics of each setting. HIV/AIDS in Latin

America falls within the framework of a low endemic setting. For the most part, the epidemic is concentrated in populations with increased risk for contracting HIV. In the countries studied, the populations identified as key groups for interventions include MSM, STI patients, CSWs, IDUs, and prisoners. Survey respondents also identified other populations with increased vulnerability for whom interventions would be crucial (e.g., young people, women). PLWHA are a priority group, since they are crucial for effective prevention interventions and can be a source of infection when access to preventive services and health care is poor.

Latin America has the necessary infrastructure and knowledge to efficiently and effectively confront the epidemic, if provided with the necessary resources. The needs vary, so it is important to adjust the interventions to respond to each country's profile and capacity. Country fact sheets provided in Appendix 1 identify the main areas for improvement and propose solutions for each country.

Given the great value added of appropriate allocation of national resources for an expanded response to the epidemic, international agencies and programs are in a position to increase regional or subregional interventions in concrete areas. Cooperation would lead to multiple returns from effective interventions, as well as to a positive cost-benefit ratio.

Results from this study show that the areas requiring the most attention for interventions in the region are as follows:

- Strengthened national HIV/AIDS programs, working collaboratively with civil societies

- Enhanced approaches focused on social mobilization and community response building

- Reduction of the risk of infection by expanding programs for the populations at highest risk (e.g., harm reduction for IDUs, counseling, condom promotion, sexual education)

- Fortified risk and vulnerability reduction programs for populations at the highest risk for infection

- Improved access to services for the populations at highest risk
- Establishment of the health care setting as a key point for prevention strategies, ensuring that PLWHA are included as target populations within prevention interventions
- Building of human capacity in different areas of expertise
- Improved capacity for monitoring and evaluation of the magnitude of the epidemic and the response
- Definition of the costs of interventions, financial gaps, and resource allocation strategies related to the response to HIV/AIDS
- Supportive legal and social norms (e.g., regarding gender, equity, human rights, stigma)
- Systematic inclusion and active engagement of PLWHA.

Country Fact Sheets

(Please note that in some countries, the prevalence rates in certain high-risk groups were not available. Therefore, they are not given.)

Mexico

HIV/AIDS Epidemic Status: Concentrated

Key HIV/AIDS Estimates

- The infection rate is greater than 5 percent in at least one high-risk group.

- Of the adult population, 0.29 percent were estimated to be living with HIV/AIDS at the end of 1999.

- A total of 150,000 people were estimated to be living with HIV/AIDS at the end of 1999.

- An estimated 4,204 people died from HIV/AIDS in 1999.

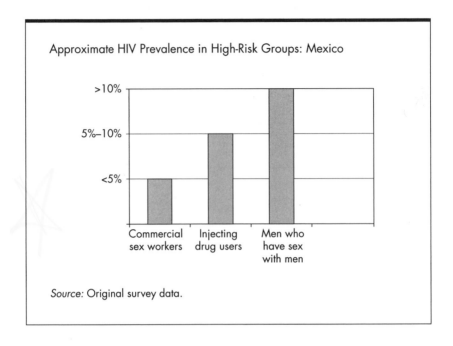

Approximate HIV Prevalence in High-Risk Groups: Mexico

Source: Original survey data.

Important Points about HIV/AIDS in Mexico

- Mexico has the third largest number of AIDS cases in the Americas, behind the United States and Brazil.

- A large proportion of migrant workers returning from the United States infect their partners.

- More rural than urban patients are female.

- Sexually transmitted infection (STI) rates are high, and rates of condom use are low.

- HIV prevalence in pregnant women was 0.6 percent in 1994 and 0.09 percent in 1996–1998.

- The most common mode of transmission is sex between men.

Funding Resources

The national HIV/AIDS program receives most of its financial support from the federal government and some from international agencies. A portion is dedicated to nongovernmental organizations (NGOs).

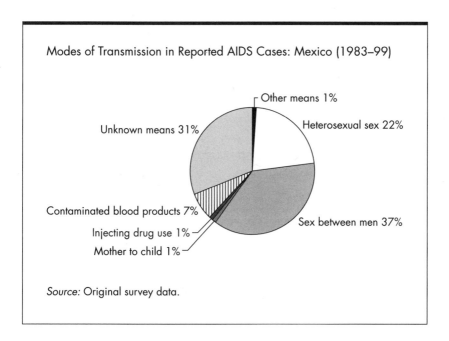

Modes of Transmission in Reported AIDS Cases: Mexico (1983–99)

Other means 1%
Heterosexual sex 22%
Unknown means 31%
Contaminated blood products 7%
Injecting drug use 1%
Mother to child 1%
Sex between men 37%

Source: Original survey data.

Prevention Issues and Challenges

Adolescents

Status: There are no adolescent-focused programs carried out in collaboration with the ministry of education.

Challenges: Sexual education and HIV/AIDS education should be introduced in the school curriculum, and interventions for high-risk adolescents are needed.

Men Who Have Sex with Men (MSM)

Status: Some programs are under way.

Challenges:

- Programs under way should be expanded in collaboration with gay-focused NGOs, states, and municipalities.

- Information and education programs should be strengthened, including education on correct condom use. Such programs should target locations frequented by MSM (e.g., saunas).

- Social, cultural, and legal barriers to homosexuality must be reduced.

Injecting Drug Users (IDUs)

Status: Current harm reduction programs offer little coverage.

Challenges:

- Programs are needed for needle exchange, promotion of HIV testing, health education, and methadone substitution. Programs should be carried out by NGOs in collaboration with the national drug program.

- The infrastructure of centers for drug addicts should be strengthened.

Prisoners

Status: Prison programs are scarce and have limited scope.

Challenges:

- Programs are needed for condom use promotion, HIV testing, and health education.

- Harm reduction programs should be planned based on needle exchange and instruction on how to clean instruments. Programs should target the prisons with the highest prevalence of IDUs.

NGO Program Funding

Challenge: Program funding should prioritize IDUs and commercial sex workers (CSWs).

Vertical Transmission

Status: Coverage of HIV testing for pregnant women is only 5 percent.

Challenges: Coverage of HIV testing for pregnant women should be expanded, and all HIV-positive pregnant women should be provided with antiretroviral therapy.

Care Issues and Challenges

Diagnosis

Status: Sixty percent of patients are diagnosed at advanced stages of infection. Access to testing is limited by lack of demand, discrimination, scarcity of health care professionals who recommend it, high cost, and scarcity of anonymous diagnosis centers.

Challenge: Anonymous diagnosis centers should be established in high-prevalence areas, and HIV testing should be promoted among MSM, CSWs, and IDUs.

Follow-up Testing

Status: Sixty-five percent of HIV/AIDS patients have had CD4 and viral load counts.

Challenge: The network of laboratories should be strengthened and expanded to increase coverage of diagnostic and monitoring tests.

Prophylaxis against Opportunistic Infections

Status: Coverage is limited; only 57 percent of patients receive this treatment.

Challenge: Continuous training in the care and treatment of HIV/AIDS patients and associated infections is needed in clinics.

Psychological and Social Support and Workplace Integration

Status: These activities have limited availability.

Challenge: Programs that respond to these needs should be organized in collaboration with self-supported NGOs and social and labor ministries.

Epidemiological Surveillance Issues and Challenges

Case Definitions, Notification Circuits, and Procedures

Status: Case definitions, notification circuits, and procedures are not defined in working protocols; thus, evaluation and corrective measures are highly labor intensive.

Challenge: National protocols for HIV and AIDS registries are needed specifying the procedures, functions, and responsibilities at each level within the surveillance system. Protocols should also include plans for periodic evaluations of the system.

Underreporting

Status: Underreporting is estimated at about 18.5 percent, with regional variations.

Challenge: HIV/AIDS case notification systems should be more exhaustive, and systems for active surveillance should be facilitated, at least in large cities.

Protection of Privacy

Status: Current legislation for protection of personal information is not extensive enough to truly guarantee confidentiality of information throughout the diagnosis and treatment process.

Challenge: Better norms are needed to ensure confidentiality of personal information.

Sentinel Surveillance

Status: Sentinel surveillance is deficient in coverage of populations (especially high-risk populations) and in procedure.

Challenge: A plan is needed for sentinel surveillance of HIV and risk factor behavior, specifying populations to monitor, methods, evaluation system, and relationship to decision making in terms of prevention activities. High-risk populations should always be prioritized.

Training

Status: Training in epidemiological surveillance has not been provided at all levels, and there is no integrated plan that consolidates information systems from the general population, sentinel sites, and other sources of information on HIV/AIDS cases.

Challenges:
- An integrated information plan is needed to monitor the epidemic through the national program and multisectorial collaborations.

- Training should be provided to all personnel responsible for epidemiological surveillance, monitoring of interventions, and multisectorial evaluation.

Blood Safety Issues and Challenges

Status: Altruistic, voluntary, and nonremunerated donations are currently combined with other forms of blood donation.

Challenge: Policies are needed to establish altruistic, voluntary, and nonremunerated donations as the only option for donation or transfusion.

Guatemala

HIV/AIDS Epidemic Status: Concentrated

Key HIV/AIDS Estimates

- The infection rate is greater than 5 percent in at least one high-risk group.

- Of the adult population, 1.4 percent were estimated to be living with HIV/AIDS at the end of 1999.

- A total of 73,000 people were estimated to be living with HIV/AIDS at the end of 1999.

- An estimated 3,600 people died from HIV/AIDS in 1999.

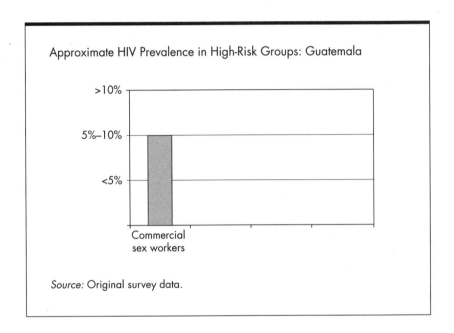

Approximate HIV Prevalence in High-Risk Groups: Guatemala

Source: Original survey data.

Important Points about HIV/AIDS in Guatemala

- The infection rate in pregnant women is less than 1 percent.

- The infection rate is up to 1.7 percent in the urban lowlands. HIV infection is still low or absent in highland regions; AIDS knowledge is very limited among indigenous highland groups and must be improved to avoid rapid spread.

Funding Resources

The national program receives support from international agencies and does not finance NGOs working with HIV/AIDS.

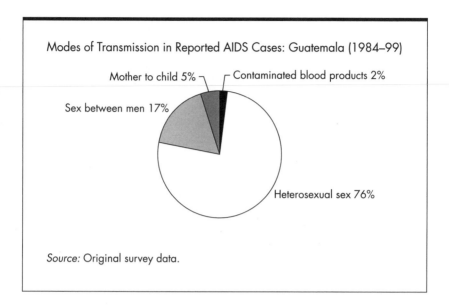

Modes of Transmission in Reported AIDS Cases: Guatemala (1984–99)

Mother to child 5% ⌐ Contaminated blood products 2%

Sex between men 17%

Heterosexual sex 76%

Source: Original survey data.

Prevention Issues and Challenges

General Population

Status: There have been few information or communication campaigns, and none thus far have promoted condom use.

Challenge: Campaigns fighting discrimination and promoting condom use should be developed and implemented.

Youths and Adolescents

Status: There are no school-based prevention programs, but rather occasional school-based activities.

Challenge: Sexual education and AIDS education should be introduced into the school curriculums in collaboration with national education authorities.

MSM

Status: Some programs are under way.

Challenge: Programs currently under way need to be expanded and coordinated with NGOs working in the large cities. Programs should focus on access to HIV testing, health education, and promotion of condom use.

CSWs

Status: Some programs are in place.

Challenge: It is necessary to expand programs for CSWs, especially in Guatemala City and other large cities. These programs should include information campaigns, promotion of HIV testing, condom distribution, and improved access and results from health centers and STI treatment and diagnosis centers.

Prisoners

Status: There is only one program in place, and coverage is low.

Challenge: More programs are needed to promote HIV testing, distribute condoms, and provide health education.

NGO Priorities

Challenge: NGOs should prioritize MSM and CSWs in their activities and maintain their current level of involvement with young people.

Vertical Transmission

Status: It is unknown how many pregnant women are offered the HIV test, and antiretroviral prophylaxis against vertical transmission is low (9 percent).

Challenge: The HIV test should be offered to all pregnant women in the most affected areas, and antiretroviral prophylaxis should be given to all HIV-positive pregnant women.

Care Issues and Challenges

Diagnosis

Status: It is not easy to obtain HIV testing. The majority of patients are diagnosed at advanced stages of infection. The main barriers to testing are the cost and social discrimination.

Challenge: Anonymous HIV diagnosis centers are needed, and testing should be promoted in high-risk groups.

Follow-up Testing

Status: Laboratory infrastructure is insufficient; only one-third of patients receive the necessary tests (only 34 percent have had CD4 and viral load counts).

Challenge: The laboratory network should be strengthened and broadened to provide more diagnostic and monitoring tests.

Social Assistance

Status: Social assistance for people affected by HIV/AIDS is limited.

Challenge: Programs should be developed to give support to PLWHA in collaboration with ministries of social affairs, labor ministries, and NGOs.

Treatment of and Prophylaxis against Opportunistic Infections

Status: There is good coverage of medications to fight opportunistic infections, but unfortunately coverage of antiretroviral treatment is low (22 percent). Sixty-four percent of patients do not take antiretrovirals because of lack of financial resources.

Challenge: Coverage of treatment of and prophylaxis against opportunistic infections should be increased.

Epidemiological Surveillance: Issues and Challenges

Case Definitions, Notification Circuits, and Procedures

Status: Case definitions, notification circuits, and procedures are not defined in working protocols; thus, evaluation and corrective measures are highly labor intensive.

Challenge: National protocols for HIV and AIDS registries are needed specifying the procedures, functions, and responsibilities at each level within the surveillance system. Protocols should also include plans for periodic evaluations of the system.

Underreporting

Status: Underreporting is estimated at about 50 percent.

Challenge: HIV/AIDS case notification systems should be more exhaustive, and systems for active surveillance are needed.

Protection of Privacy

Status: Current legislation for protection of personal information is not extensive enough to truly guarantee confidentiality of information throughout the diagnosis and treatment process.

Challenge: Better norms are needed to ensure confidentiality of personal information.

Sentinel Surveillance

Status: Sentinel surveillance is deficient in coverage of populations (especially high-risk populations) and in procedure.

Challenge: A plan is needed for sentinel surveillance of HIV and risk factor behavior, specifying populations to monitor, methods, evaluation system, and relationship to decision making in terms of prevention activities. High-risk populations should always be prioritized.

Training

Status: Training in epidemiological surveillance has not been provided at all levels, and there is no integrated plan that consolidates information systems from the general population, sentinel sites, and other sources of information on HIV/AIDS cases.

Challenges:
- An integrated information plan is needed to monitor the epidemic, through the national program and multisectorial collaborations.

- Training should be provided to all personnel responsible for epidemiological surveillance, monitoring of interventions, and multisectorial evaluation.

Blood Safety Issues and Challenges

Status: Altruistic, voluntary, and nonremunerated donations are currently combined with other forms of blood donation.

Challenge: Policies are needed to establish altruistic, voluntary, and nonremunerated donations as the only option for donation or transfusion.

El Salvador

HIV/AIDS Epidemic Status: Concentrated

Key HIV/AIDS Estimates
- The infection rate is greater than 5 percent in at least one high-risk group.

- Of the adult population, 0.6 percent were estimated to be living with HIV/AIDS at the end of 1999.

- A total of 20,000 people were estimated to be living with HIV/AIDS at the end of 1999.

- An estimated 1,300 people died from HIV/AIDS in 1999.

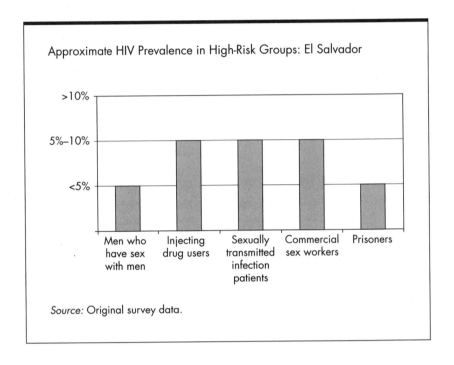

Approximate HIV Prevalence in High-Risk Groups: El Salvador

Source: Original survey data.

Important Points about HIV/AIDS in El Salvador

- Seventy-five percent of reported cases are from San Salvador.

- The infection rate in pregnant women is less than 1 percent.

- HIV prevalence in women of childbearing age is 0.5 percent (0–1.1 percent).

- In blood donors HIV prevalence was 0.13 percent in 1996–97.

- The major mode of transmission is heterosexual sex.

Funding Resources

The national HIV/AIDS program does not receive support from international agencies and does not finance NGOs.

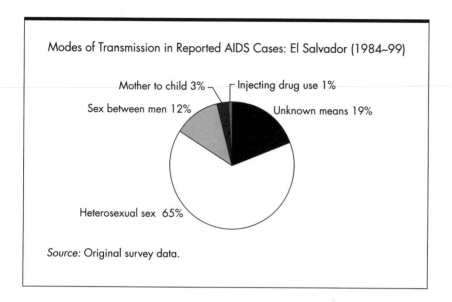

Modes of Transmission in Reported AIDS Cases: El Salvador (1984–99)

Mother to child 3% — Injecting drug use 1%

Sex between men 12% — Unknown means 19%

Heterosexual sex 65%

Source: Original survey data.

Prevention Issues and Challenges

General Population

Status: There have been few campaigns for the general population, and very few have focused on condom promotion.

Challenge: Campaigns fighting discrimination and promoting condom use should be developed.

Adolescents

Status: There is no plan in the ministry of health for including sexual education or AIDS education in the school curriculums.

Challenge: In collaboration with the ministry of health, sexual education and AIDS and drug education programs should be initiated in schools, beginning in the areas with highest HIV prevalence.

MSM

Status: There are no programs for MSM, only occasional activities.

Challenge: A national strategy for interventions targeting MSM should be designed in collaboration with the national and local gay movements. The majority of NGO programs should prioritize MSM.

CSWs

Status: Some programs are under way.

Challenge: It is necessary to expand programs for CSWs, especially in the large cities. These programs should include information campaigns, promotion of HIV testing, condom distribution, and improved access and results from health centers and sexually transmitted infection (STI) treatment and diagnosis centers.

Prisoners

Status: There is only one program for prisoners, which offers little coverage.

Challenge: The existing program should be expanded, and more programs should be developed to promote access to HIV testing and STI diagnosis and provide health education.

NGO Priorities

Challenge: NGO programs should prioritize MSM and CSWs.

Vertical Transmission

Status: It is unknown how many pregnant women are offered HIV testing or how many received antiretroviral prophylaxis.

Challenge: HIV testing should be offered to all pregnant women in the most affected regions, and antiretroviral prophylaxis should be given to all HIV-positive pregnant women.

Care Issues and Challenges

Diagnosis

Status: It is not easy to get HIV testing. Sixty percent of patients diagnosed with HIV presented at advanced stages of infection. The main barriers to testing are cost and social discrimination.

Challenge: Anonymous diagnosis centers should be established, and HIV testing should be promoted in high-risk populations.

Follow-up Testing

Status: Half of HIV/AIDS patients have had a CD4 count, and only 4 percent have had a viral load count.

Challenge: The network of laboratories providing these tests should be strengthened and expanded to provide greater coverage of diagnostic and monitoring tests.

Social Support and Workplace Integration

Status: Social support and workplace integration activities are still weak.

Challenge: Community self-help initiatives, as well as social programs for PLWHA, should be promoted in collaboration with social and labor ministries.

Treatment

Status: Coverage of antiretroviral treatment is low (14 percent). Fifty-two percent of HIV/AIDS patients are not on antiretroviral therapy because they lack financial resources.

Challenge: Increase coverage of antiretroviral treatment.

Epidemiological Surveillance Issues and Challenges

Case Definitions, Notification Circuits, and Procedures

Status: Case definitions, notification circuits, and procedures are not defined in working protocols; thus, evaluation and corrective measures are highly labor intensive.

Challenge: National protocols for HIV and AIDS registries are needed specifying the procedures, functions, and responsibilities at each level within the surveillance system. Protocols should also include plans for periodic evaluations of the system.

Underreporting

Status: Underreporting is estimated at about 40 percent.

Challenge: HIV/AIDS case notification systems should be more exhaustive, and systems for active surveillance are needed.

Protection of Privacy

Status: Current legislation for protection of personal information is not extensive enough to truly guarantee confidentiality of information throughout the diagnosis and treatment process.

Challenge: Better norms are needed to ensure confidentiality of personal information.

Sentinel Surveillance

Status: Sentinel surveillance is deficient in coverage of populations (especially high-risk populations) and in procedure.

Challenge: A plan is needed for sentinel surveillance of HIV and risk factor behavior, specifying populations to monitor, methods, evaluation system, and relationship to decision making in terms of prevention activities. High-risk populations should always be prioritized.

Training

Status: Training in epidemiological surveillance has not been provided at all levels, and there is no integrated plan that consolidates information systems from the general population, sentinel sites, and other sources of information on HIV/AIDS cases.

Challenges:
- An integrated information plan is needed to monitor the epidemic, through the national program and multisectorial collaborations.

- Training should be provided to all personnel responsible for epidemiological surveillance, monitoring of interventions, and multisectorial evaluation.

Case Reporting

Status: Cases are reported by clinicians, and also by people outside the medical field.

Challenge: Norms are needed to delegate case notification responsibilities exclusively to health care personnel (clinicians or laboratory personnel).

Blood Safety Issues and Challenges

Status: Altruistic, voluntary, and nonremunerated donations are currently combined with other forms of blood donation.

Challenge: Policies are needed to establish altruistic, voluntary, and nonremunerated donations as the only option for donation or transfusion.

Honduras

HIV/AIDS Epidemic Status: Generalized

- Of the adult population, 1.9 percent were estimated to be living with HIV/AIDS at the end of 1999.

- A total of 63,000 people were estimated to be living with HIV/ AIDS at the end of 1999.

- An estimated 4,200 people died from HIV/AIDS in 1999.

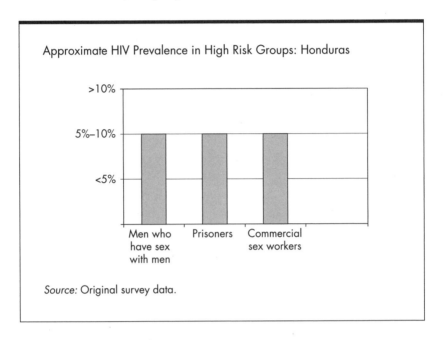

Approximate HIV Prevalence in High Risk Groups: Honduras

Source: Original survey data.

Important Points about HIV/AIDS in Honduras

- Honduras has the highest prevalence of HIV in Latin America.

- Nearly as many females as males are infected, and AIDS is the leading cause of death among women of childbearing age.

- The HIV infection rate among Garífunas is six times the national average.

- HIV prevalence in pregnant women is 1.4 percent overall and 2–5 percent in San Pedro Sula.

- HIV prevalence among blood donors is 0.6 percent in Tegucigalpa and 1.0 percent in San Pedro Sula.

- The most common mode of transmission is heterosexual sex.

Funding Resources

The national HIV/AIDS program receives support from international agencies and finances NGOs.

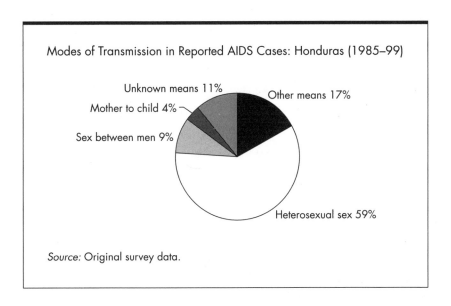

Modes of Transmission in Reported AIDS Cases: Honduras (1985–99)

Unknown means 11%
Mother to child 4%
Sex between men 9%
Other means 17%
Heterosexual sex 59%

Source: Original survey data.

Prevention Issues and Challenges

General Population

Status: Some campaigns are under way.

Challenge: More campaigns fighting discrimination and promoting condom use should be implemented.

Youths and Adolescents

Status: Coverage of sexual education and AIDS education programs is about 50 percent in public schools.

Challenges:

- Coverage of school-based programs should be increased, especially in the most affected cities.

- Efforts should be focused on high-risk adolescents, as well as those who do not attend school.

MSM

Status: Programs are in place, but coverage is low.

Challenge: Current programs should be strengthened and expanded in collaboration with MSM-focused NGOs. Information, health education, and instruction on condom use should be emphasized, and these programs should reach out to MSM in their communities.

CSWs

Status: Some programs are under way.

Challenge: Programs for CSWs should be expanded in large cities. These programs should include information campaigns, promotion of HIV testing, condom distribution, and improved access and results from health centers and STI treatment and diagnosis centers.

Prisoners

Status: There are currently no programs for prisoners.

Challenge: Interventions for prisoners should be designed and implemented focusing on health education, condom distribution, and access to health services and STI and HIV diagnosis.

NGO Funding

Challenge: Funding allocated to NGOs should prioritize those with interventions for MSM and CSWs.

Vertical Transmission

Status: Very few pregnant women are offered HIV testing (8 percent), and very few HIV-positive pregnant women receive antiretroviral prophylaxis (20 percent).

Challenge: All pregnant women in the most affected areas should be offered HIV testing, and antiretroviral prophylaxis should be provided to all HIV-positive pregnant women.

Care Issues and Challenges

Diagnosis

Status: It is not easy to obtain HIV testing because of social discrimination, cost, and the infrequency of health care professionals recommending or offering the test. Sixty percent of patients diagnosed with HIV present at advanced stages of infection.

Challenges:
- Anonymous diagnosis centers should be established, and HIV testing should be promoted in high-risk populations.

- Symptomatic management of STIs should be expanded, and HIV testing should be more frequent in patients presenting with suspected STIs.

Follow-up Testing

Status: Very few HIV/AIDS patients have had CD4 or viral load counts (only 3 percent), and the laboratory network is not capable of providing the necessary coverage.

Challenge: The network of laboratories providing these tests should be strengthened and expanded to provide greater coverage of diagnostic and monitoring tests.

Treatment

Status: Eighty-six percent of HIV/AIDS patients are not on anti-retroviral therapy because they lack financial resources, and only 3 percent of HIV/AIDS patients are on highly active antiretroviral therapy (HAART).

Challenge: There is a great need for training for health care professionals in clinical management and treatment of HIV/AIDS patients.

Psychological and Social Support and Workplace Integration

Status: Activities are still weak.

Challenge: Community self-help initiatives should be promoted, as well as social programs for people living with HIV/AIDS, in collaboration with social and labor ministries.

Epidemiological Surveillance Issues and Challenges

Case Definitions, Notification Circuits, and Procedures

Status: Case definitions, notification circuits, and procedures are not defined in working protocols; thus, evaluation and corrective measures are highly labor intensive.

Challenge: National protocols for HIV and AIDS registries are needed specifying the procedures, functions, and responsibilities at each level within the surveillance system. Protocols should also include plans for periodic evaluations of the system.

Underreporting

Status: Underreporting is estimated at about 47 percent.

Challenge: HIV/AIDS case notification systems should be more exhaustive, and systems for active surveillance are needed.

Protection of Privacy

Status: Current legislation for protection of personal information is not extensive enough to truly guarantee confidentiality of information throughout the diagnosis and treatment process.

Challenge: Better norms are needed to ensure confidentiality of personal information.

Sentinel Surveillance

Status: Sentinel surveillance is deficient in coverage of populations (especially high-risk populations) and in procedure.

Challenge: A plan is needed for sentinel surveillance of HIV and risk factor behavior, specifying populations to monitor, methods, evaluation system, and relationship to decision making in terms of prevention activities. High-risk populations should always be prioritized.

Training

Status: Training in epidemiological surveillance has not been provided at all levels, and there is no integrated plan that consolidates information systems from the general population, sentinel sites, and other sources of information on HIV/AIDS cases.

Challenges:
- An integrated information plan is needed to monitor the epidemic, through the national program and multisectorial collaborations.

- Training should be provided to all personnel responsible for epidemiological surveillance, monitoring of interventions, and multisectorial evaluation.

Case Reporting

Status: Cases are reported by clinicians and also by people outside the medical field.

Challenge: Norms are needed to delegate case notification responsibilities exclusively to health care personnel (clinicians or laboratory personnel).

Blood Safety Issues and Challenges

Status: Altruistic, voluntary, and nonremunerated donations are currently combined with other forms of blood donation.

Challenge: Policies are needed to establish altruistic, voluntary, and nonremunerated donations as the only option for donation or transfusion.

Nicaragua

HIV/AIDS Epidemic Status: Low Level

Key HIV/AIDS Estimates

- The infection rate is less than 5 percent in high-risk groups.
- Of the adult population, 0.2 percent were estimated to be living with HIV/AIDS at the end of 1999.
- A total of 4,900 people were estimated to be living with HIV/AIDS at the end of 1999.
- An estimated 360 people died from HIV/AIDS in 1999.

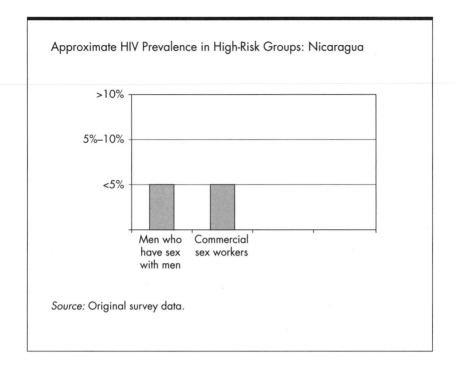

Approximate HIV Prevalence in High-Risk Groups: Nicaragua

Source: Original survey data.

Important Points about HIV/AIDS in Nicaragua

• More than 50 percent of reported AIDS cases are from Managua.

• No surveillance data on HIV prevalence in pregnant women are available.

• Gonorrhea and syphilis rates are high; reported condom use is low.

• The infection rate in blood donors is 0.05–0.09 percent.

• The most common mode of transmission is heterosexual sex.

Funding Resources

The national HIV/AIDS program receives support from international agencies and finances NGOs.

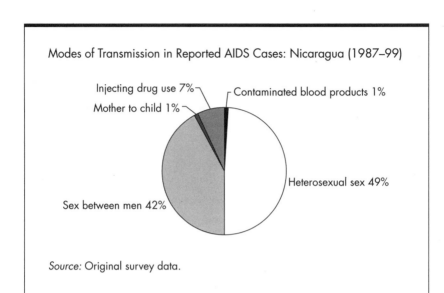

Modes of Transmission in Reported AIDS Cases: Nicaragua (1987–99)

Injecting drug use 7%

Mother to child 1%

Contaminated blood products 1%

Heterosexual sex 49%

Sex between men 42%

Source: Original survey data.

Prevention Issues and Challenges

Youths and Adolescents

Status: Formal education coverage is very low (32 percent).

Challenge: Programs for adolescents attending school should be expanded, and programs should be started or expanded for high-risk adolescents and those who do not attend school.

MSM

Status: Some programs are under way.

Challenge: It is necessary to expand programs for MSM in large cities. Toll-free information hotlines may facilitate this.

CSWs

Status: Some programs are under way.

Challenge: It is necessary to expand programs for CSWs, especially in large cities.

Prisoners

Status: Programs for prisoners are fairly new and offer little coverage.

Challenge: These programs should be expanded to cover more prisoners and should include condom distribution and health education.

Care Issues and Challenges

Diagnosis

Status: Almost all HIV/AIDS patients are diagnosed at the point of advanced infection or full-blown AIDS. HIV testing is free in some health centers.

Challenges:
- Eliminate the main barriers to testing: Professionals often do not offer the test, and social discrimination discourages access.
- To facilitate earlier detection, HIV testing should be promoted and should be made more available in health centers.

Follow-up Testing

Status: The network of laboratories offering CD4 and viral load counts is insufficient. Less than 1 percent of HIV/AIDS patients have had a CD4 or viral load count.

Challenge: It is necessary to broaden the services offered by laboratories.

Treatment

Status: Seventy-two percent of patients do not take antiretrovirals because they lack the financial resources, and only 3 percent of HIV/AIDS patients are on HAART.

Challenge: Improve the percentage of patients receiving the treatment they need.

Psychological and Social Support and Workplace Integration

Status: Coverage of these activities is low.

Challenge: Resources should be increased so that health centers and NGOs can provide more psychological and social services.

Epidemiological Surveillance Issues and Challenges

Case Definitions, Notification Circuits, and Procedures

Status: Case definitions, notification circuits, and procedures are not defined in working protocols; thus, evaluation and corrective measures are highly labor intensive.

Challenge: National protocols for HIV and AIDS registries are needed specifying the procedures, functions, and responsibilities at each level within the surveillance system. Protocols should also include plans for periodic evaluations of the system.

Underreporting

Status: Underreporting is estimated at about 60 percent.

Challenge: HIV/AIDS case notification systems should be more exhaustive, and systems for active surveillance are needed.

Protection of Privacy

Status: Current legislation for protection of personal information is not extensive enough to truly guarantee confidentiality of information throughout the diagnosis and treatment process.

Challenge: Better norms are needed to ensure confidentiality of personal information.

Sentinel Surveillance

Status: Sentinel surveillance is deficient in coverage of populations (especially high-risk populations) and in procedure.

Challenge: A plan is needed for sentinel surveillance of HIV and risk factor behavior, specifying populations to monitor, methods, evaluation system, and relationship to decision making in terms of prevention activities. High-risk populations should always be prioritized.

Training

Status: Training in epidemiological surveillance has not been provided at all levels, and there is no integrated plan that consolidates information systems from the general population, sentinel sites, and other sources of information on HIV/AIDS cases.

Challenges:
- An integrated information plan is needed to monitor the epidemic through the national program and multisectorial collaborations.
- Training should be provided to all personnel responsible for epidemiological surveillance, monitoring interventions, and multisectorial evaluation.

Blood Safety Issues and Challenges

Status: Altruistic, voluntary, and nonremunerated donations are currently combined with other forms of blood donation.

Challenge: Policies are needed to establish altruistic, voluntary, and nonremunerated donations as the only option for donation or transfusion.

Costa Rica

HIV/AIDS Epidemic Status: Concentrated

Key HIV/AIDS Estimates

- The infection rate is less than 5 percent in high-risk groups.

- Of the adult population, 0.53 percent were estimated to be living with HIV/AIDS at the end of 1999.

- A total of 12,000 people were estimated to be living with HIV/AIDS at the end of 1999.

- An estimated 750 people died from HIV/AIDS in 1999.

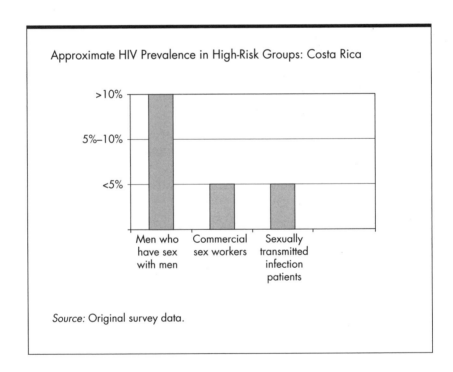

Approximate HIV Prevalence in High-Risk Groups: Costa Rica

Source: Original survey data.

Important Points about HIV/AIDS in Costa Rica

- Universal social security provides HIV/AIDS care, including anti-retroviral therapy, to all.

- HIV/AIDS infections are concentrated in urban zones.

- Costa Rica is unique in Central America for the predominance of MSM among reported AIDS cases.

- HIV prevalence in pregnant women is less than 0.5 percent.

Funding Resources

The national HIV/AIDS program receives support from international agencies and does not finance NGOs.

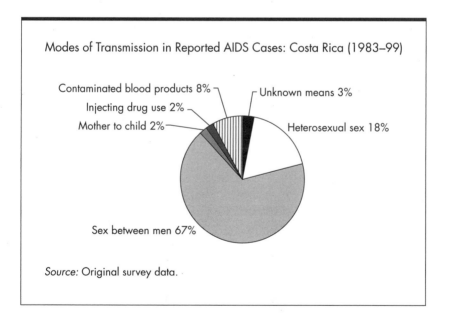

Modes of Transmission in Reported AIDS Cases: Costa Rica (1983–99)

Contaminated blood products 8%

Unknown means 3%

Injecting drug use 2%

Mother to child 2%

Heterosexual sex 18%

Sex between men 67%

Source: Original survey data.

Prevention Issues and Challenges

General Population

Status: Information and prevention campaigns have been scarce, and none have promoted condom use.

Challenge: More campaigns should be carried out for the general population and youths focusing on promoting condom use.

Youths and Adolescents

Status: There are currently no school-based programs.

Challenge: Sexual education and HIV/AIDS education should be incorporated into school curriculums, in collaboration with national education authorities.

MSM

Status: There are currently no programs for MSM, but rather occasional activities.

Challenges:
- A national strategy for MSM initiatives should be designed in collaboration with the national and local gay movements.

- NGO programs should prioritize MSM.

CSWs

Status: Only occasional activities have been carried out, and there have been no interventions for male CSWs or transvestites.

Challenge: It is necessary to develop a program including information campaigns, promotion of HIV testing, condom distribution, and improved access and results from health centers and STI treatment and diagnosis centers.

Prisoners

Status: Some programs are under way.

Challenge: More interventions for prisoners should be designed and implemented focusing on health education, condom distribution, and access to health services and STI and HIV testing and diagnosis.

Vertical Transmission

Status: Universal testing is recommended for all pregnant women, but actual coverage is unknown.

Challenge: Evaluations of the rate at which testing is offered and carried out should be conducted, and HIV testing should be offered more frequently.

Condom Access

Status: Access to condoms is limited.

Challenge: More condoms should be available at pharmacies and supermarkets, areas frequented by MSM, education centers, and universities.

Care Issues and Challenges

Treatment

Status: Health care and treatment coverage is very high.

Challenge: Programs are needed to train health care professionals in clinical management of HIV/AIDS patients and administration of antiretroviral therapies.

Psychological and Social Support and Workplace Integration

Status: Social support and workplace integration activities are still weak.

Challenge: Self-supported community initiatives should be promoted, as well as social programs for PLWHA in collaboration with social and labor ministries.

Epidemiological Surveillance Issues and Challenges

Case Definitions, Notification Circuits, and Procedures

Status: Case definitions, notification circuits, and procedures are not defined in working protocols; thus, evaluation and corrective measures are highly labor intensive.

Challenge: National protocols for HIV and AIDS registries are needed specifying the procedures, functions, and responsibilities at each level within the surveillance system. Protocols should also include plans for periodic evaluations of the system.

Underreporting

Status: Underreporting is estimated at about 50 percent.

Challenge: HIV/AIDS case notification systems should be more exhaustive, and systems for active surveillance are needed.

Protection of Privacy

Status: Current legislation for protection of personal information is not extensive enough to truly guarantee confidentiality of information throughout the diagnosis and treatment process.

Challenge: Better norms are needed to ensure confidentiality of personal information.

Sentinel Surveillance

Status: Sentinel surveillance is deficient in coverage of populations (especially high-risk populations) and in procedure.

Challenge: A plan is needed for sentinel surveillance of HIV and risk factor behavior, specifying populations to monitor, methods, evaluation system, and relationship to decision making in terms of prevention activities. High-risk populations should always be prioritized.

Training

Status: Training in epidemiological surveillance has not been provided at all levels, and there is no integrated plan that consolidates information systems from the general population, sentinel sites, and other sources of information on HIV/AIDS cases.

Challenges:

- An integrated information plan is needed to monitor the epidemic through the national program and multisectorial collaborations.

- Training should be provided to all personnel responsible for epidemiological surveillance, monitoring of interventions, and multisectorial evaluation.

Blood Safety Issues and Challenges

Status: Altruistic, voluntary, and nonremunerated donations are currently combined with other forms of blood donation.

Challenge: Policies are needed to establish altruistic, voluntary, and nonremunerated donations as the only option for donation or transfusion.

Panama

HIV/AIDS Epidemic Status: Low Level

Key HIV/AIDS Estimates

- The infection rate is less than 5 percent in high-risk groups.

- Of the adult population, 1.5 percent were estimated to be living with HIV/AIDS at the end of 1999.

- A total of 24,000 people were estimated to be living with HIV/AIDS at the end of 1999.

- An estimated 1,200 people died from HIV/AIDS in 1999.

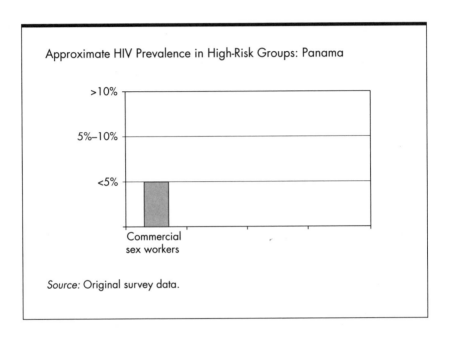

Approximate HIV Prevalence in High-Risk Groups: Panama

Commercial sex workers

Source: Original survey data.

Important Points about HIV/AIDS in Panama

- Panama has the second-highest HIV/AIDS rate in Central America, but surveillance data from high-risk groups is lacking.

- HIV infection and STIs are increasing.

- Of the prison population, 5.8 percent were reported HIV positive in 1991.

- HIV prevalence in pregnant women was up to 0.9 percent in 1997.

- The most common mode of transmission is heterosexual sex.

Funding Resources

The national HIV/AIDS program receives financial support from international agencies and does not finance national NGOs. Panama's national program is the newest HIV/AIDS national program in Latin America, and it has not yet articulated an integrated national response.

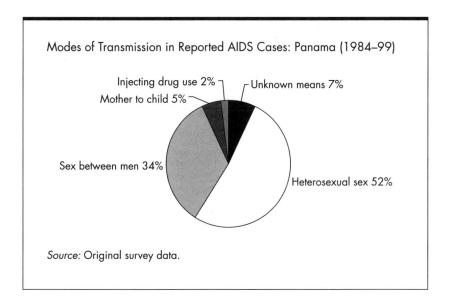

Modes of Transmission in Reported AIDS Cases: Panama (1984–99)

Injecting drug use 2%
Mother to child 5%
Unknown means 7%
Sex between men 34%
Heterosexual sex 52%

Source: Original survey data.

Prevention Issues and Challenges

General Population

Status: Prevention and information campaigns have been insufficient.

Challenge: More campaigns promoting condom use among youths are needed.

Youths and Adolescents

Status: There are no school-based prevention programs.

Challenges:
- Sexual education and HIV/AIDS education should be introduced in the school curriculum in collaboration with national education authorities.

- Health education programs specifically targeting high-risk adolescents should be developed.

MSM

Status: There are no programs for MSM.

Challenges:
- A national strategy for MSM interventions should be designed in collaboration with the national or local gay movements.

- NGO programs should prioritize MSM.

CSWs

Status: There are no programs for CSWs. Health care control is obligatory, but individuals must pay for services.

Challenges:
- A program is needed to provide information, promote HIV testing, and distribute condoms to CSWs, as well as to improve and expand access to health centers and STI centers where free services could be obtained.

- NGOs working with street workers should be supported.

Prisoners

Status: A program for prisoners is under way but offers little coverage.

Challenge: This program should be expanded to promote access to HIV testing, STI diagnosis, and condom distribution.

Vertical Transmission

Status: It is unknown how many pregnant women are offered the HIV test or how many received antiretroviral prophylaxis.

Challenge: Coverage of HIV testing for pregnant women should be evaluated, and access to prophylaxis for HIV-positive pregnant women should be promoted.

Access to Condoms

Status: Condoms are available only in pharmacies and supermarkets.

Challenge: Condoms should be available in more locations, especially places where CSWs and MSM frequent, as well as in youth and education centers.

Community Movements and NGOs

Status: Community and NGO involvement with HIV/AIDS is scarce.

Challenge: Community responses need to be strengthened, and NGOs should be supported and new ones introduced.

Care Issues and Challenges

Diagnosis

Status: Barriers to HIV testing include scarcity of demand and discrimination.

Challenge: Anonymous diagnosis centers should be expanded, and the HIV test should be offered in STI diagnosis and treatment centers.

Follow-up Testing

Status: Coverage of laboratory tests is limited. Only 24 percent of HIV/AIDS patients have had CD4 and viral load counts.

Challenge: The network of laboratories providing these tests should be strengthened and expanded.

Prophylaxis against Opportunistic Infections

Status: Coverage of prophylaxis against opportunistic infections is low (45 percent).

Challenge: Continuous training in the management of HIV/AIDS patients is needed in clinics. This training should include current recommendations for prophylactic measures and antiretroviral therapies.

Epidemiological Surveillance Issues and Challenges

Case Definitions, Notification Circuits, and Procedures

Status: Case definitions, notification circuits, and procedures are not defined in working protocols; thus, evaluation and corrective measures are highly labor intensive.

Challenge: National protocols for HIV and AIDS registries are needed specifying the procedures, functions, and responsibilities at each level within the surveillance system. Protocols should also include plans for periodic evaluations of the system.

Underreporting

Status: Underreporting is estimated at about 32 percent.

Challenge: HIV/AIDS case notification systems should be more exhaustive, and systems for active surveillance are needed.

Protection of Privacy

Status: Current legislation for protection of personal information is not extensive enough to truly guarantee confidentiality of information throughout the diagnosis and treatment process.

Challenge: Better norms are needed to ensure confidentiality of personal information.

Sentinel Surveillance

Status: Sentinel surveillance is deficient in coverage of populations (especially high-risk populations) and in procedure.

Challenge: A plan is needed for sentinel surveillance of HIV and risk factor behavior, specifying populations to monitor, methods, evaluation system, and relationship to decision making in terms of prevention activities. High-risk populations should always be prioritized.

Training

Status: Training in epidemiological surveillance has not been provided at all levels, and there is no integrated plan that consolidates information systems from the general population, sentinel sites, and other sources of information on HIV/AIDS cases.

Challenges:
- An integrated information plan is needed to monitor the epidemic through the national program and multisectorial collaborations.

- Training should be provided to all personnel responsible for epidemiological surveillance, monitoring interventions, and multisectorial evaluation.

Case Reporting

Status: Cases are reported by clinicians and also by people outside the medical field.

Challenge: Norms are needed to delegate case notification responsibilities exclusively to health care personnel (clinicians or laboratory personnel).

Blood Safety Issues and Challenges

Status: Altruistic, voluntary, and nonremunerated donations are currently combined with other forms of blood donation.

Challenge: Policies are needed to establish altruistic, voluntary, and non-remunerated donations as the only option for donation or transfusion.

Brazil

HIV/AIDS Epidemic Status: Concentrated

Key HIV/AIDS Estimates

- The infection rate is greater than 5 percent in at least one high-risk group.

- Of the adult population, 0.60 percent were estimated to be living with HIV/AIDS at the end of 1999.

- A total of 540,000 people were estimated to be living with HIV/AIDS at the end of 1999.

- An estimated 18,000 people died from HIV/AIDS in 1999.

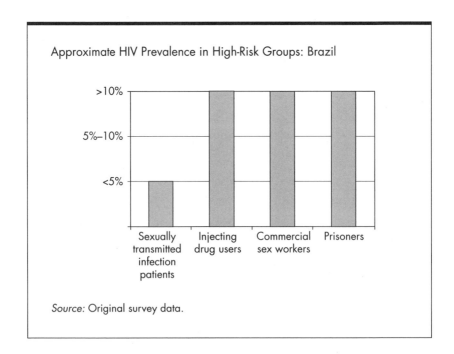

Approximate HIV Prevalence in High-Risk Groups: Brazil

Source: Original survey data.

Important Points about HIV/AIDS in Brazil

- Brazil has the second largest number of AIDS cases in the Americas, behind the United States.

- Injecting drug use is increasing in importance as a route of HIV transmission.

- The epidemic is concentrated in the southeast but is spreading to the northeast.

- Locally produced generic antiretroviral medications are provided by the government to people living with HIV/AIDS.

- HIV prevalence in pregnant women was 0.6–1.5 percent (2.6–3.3 percent in Porto Alegre) in 1996–97.

- The major mode of transmission is sex between men.

Funding Resources

The country receives financial support from international agencies and finances NGOs.

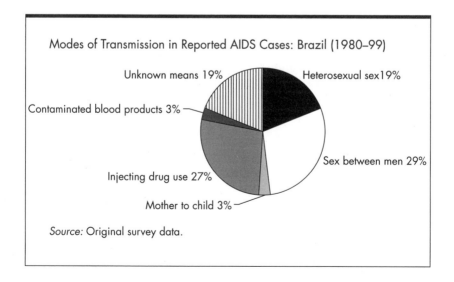

Modes of Transmission in Reported AIDS Cases: Brazil (1980–99)

Unknown means 19%
Heterosexual sex 19%
Contaminated blood products 3%
Sex between men 29%
Injecting drug use 27%
Mother to child 3%

Source: Original survey data.

Prevention Issues and Challenges

MSM

Status: Prevalence among MSM is high. Some programs are under way.

Challenges:
- Programs already in place should be expanded in collaboration with gay-focused NGOs, states, and municipalities.

- Information and education programs should be strengthened, including education on correct condom use. Such programs should target locations frequented by MSM (e.g., saunas).

CSWs

Status: Some programs in place, with limited coverage.

Challenge: Coverage of programs needs to be expanded, including programs for male CSWs. NGO programs should prioritize CSWs working on streets and in clubs.

IDUs

Status: Current harm reduction programs have recently started and offer limited coverage.

Challenge: Needle exchange programs are needed, especially through outreach programs. Pharmacists and health centers should be involved in needle exchange programs in order to increase coverage.

Prisoners

Status: Prison programs have recently begun, and rates of HIV infection are high.

Challenges:
- Programs for prisoners need to include promotion of HIV testing, diagnosis and treatment of sexually transmitted infections (STIs), and health education.

- Harm reduction programs should be planned based on needle exchange and instruction on how to clean instruments. These programs should target the prisons with the highest prevalence of IDUs and should be coordinated with services provided outside prisons to ensure continuity.

Vertical Transmission

Status: Only half of pregnant women are offered HIV testing, and only 40 percent of HIV-positive pregnant women receive antiretroviral prophylaxis.

Challenge: HIV testing should be offered to all pregnant women, and antiretroviral prophylaxis should be increased for HIV-positive pregnant women.

Care Issues and Challenges

Diagnosis

Status: Seventy-five percent of patients are diagnosed at advanced stages of infection or when they have already progressed to AIDS.

Challenge: In order to promote early diagnosis, testing should be promoted through the creation and expansion of anonymous diagnosis centers and programs for high-risk groups, including people with STIs.

Follow-up Testing

Status: Only 8 percent of patients had had CD4 and viral load counts. The laboratory network is limited in terms of coverage in states and municipalities.

Challenge: The network of laboratories should be strengthened, and new laboratories should be incorporated to increase the availability of CD4 and viral load tests.

Prophylaxis against Opportunistic Infections

Status: Coverage is very low (13 percent).

Challenge: Continuous training is needed in the management and treatment of HIV/AIDS patients in accordance with current norms and standards.

Treatment

Status: A substantial proportion of HIV positive patients (85 percent by government estimate) who have indications for antiretroviral treatment receive HAART.

Psychological and Social Support and Workplace Integration

Status: These activities have limited availability.

Challenge: In collaboration with NGOs and social and labor ministries, programs should be organized to improve social and psychological care in some areas.

Epidemiological Surveillance Issues and Challenges

Case Definitions, Notification Circuits, and Procedures

Status: Case definitions, notification circuits, and procedures are not defined in working protocols; thus, evaluation and corrective measures are highly labor intensive.

Challenge: National protocols for HIV and AIDS registries are needed specifying the procedures, functions, and responsibilities at each level within the surveillance system. Protocols should also include plans for periodic evaluations of the system.

Underreporting

Status: Underreporting is estimated at about 5 percent to 10 percent, but it may be even higher.

Challenge: HIV/AIDS case notification systems should be more exhaustive, and already existing systems for active surveillance should be facilitated.

Protection of Privacy

Status: Current legislation for protection of personal information is not extensive enough to truly guarantee confidentiality of information throughout the diagnosis and treatment process.

Challenge: Better norms are needed to ensure confidentiality of personal information.

Sentinel Surveillance

Status: Sentinel surveillance is deficient in coverage of populations (especially high-risk populations) and in procedure.

Challenge: A plan is needed for sentinel surveillance of HIV and risk factor behavior, specifying populations to monitor, methods, evaluation system, and relationship to decision making in terms of prevention activities. High-risk populations should always be prioritized.

Training

Status: Training in epidemiological surveillance has not been provided at all levels, and there is no integrated plan that consolidates information systems from the general population, sentinel sites, and other sources of information on HIV/AIDS cases.

Challenges:
- An integrated information plan is needed to monitor the epidemic through the national program and multisectorial collaborations.

- Training should be provided to all personnel responsible for epidemiological surveillance, monitoring interventions, and multisectorial evaluation.

HIV/AIDS Registry

Status: There has been increased access to antiretroviral treatment and the reduction in AIDS cases and mortality.

Challenge: A universal registry of HIV infection should be created.

Blood Safety Issues and Challenges

Status: Altruistic, voluntary, and nonremunerated donations are currently combined with other forms of blood donation.

Challenge: Policies are needed to establish altruistic, voluntary, and nonremunerated donations as the only option for donation or transfusion.

República Bolivariana de Venezuela

HIV/AIDS Epidemic Status: Low Level

Key HIV/AIDS Estimates

- The infection rate is less than 5 percent in high-risk groups.

- Of the adult population, 0.49 percent were estimated to be living with HIV/AIDS at the end of 1999.

- A total of 62,000 people were estimated to be living with HIV/AIDS at the end of 1999.

- An estimated 2,000 people died from HIV/AIDS in 1999.

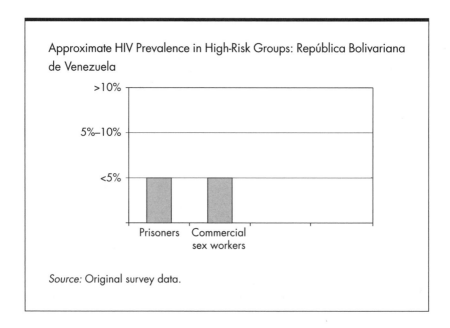

Approximate HIV Prevalence in High-Risk Groups: República Bolivariana de Venezuela

Source: Original survey data.

Important Points about HIV/AIDS in the República Bolivariana de Venezuela

- Little information about the HIV/AIDS epidemic in the República Bolivariana de Venezuela is available; data suggest the epidemic may be more advanced than official statistics indicate.

- HIV is believed to be increasing in tourist, industrial, and mining areas.

- The highest HIV prevalence is reported from Caribbean islands (e.g., Margarita Island).

- HIV prevalence in pregnant women was 0.0 percent in 1996.

- The most common mode of transmission is sex between men.

Funding Resources

The national program receives support from international agencies and does not finance NGOs.

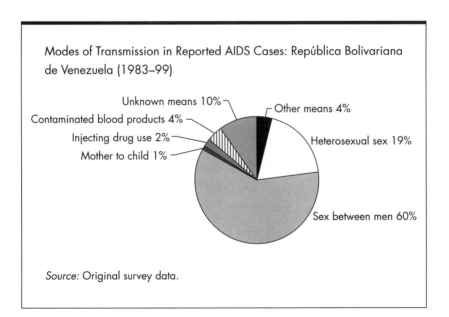

Modes of Transmission in Reported AIDS Cases: República Bolivariana de Venezuela (1983–99)

Unknown means 10%
Contaminated blood products 4%
Injecting drug use 2%
Mother to child 1%
Other means 4%
Heterosexual sex 19%
Sex between men 60%

Source: Original survey data.

Prevention Issues and Challenges

Adolescents

Status: Some programs are under way.

Challenge: Programs are needed for high-risk adolescents. Such programs should be extended in the main urban areas.

MSM

Status: Some programs are under way.

Challenges:
- Programs already under way should be expanded and coordinated with NGOs in large cities.
- Programs should be based on increasing access to HIV testing, health education, and promotion of condom use.

IDUs

Status: There are currently no programs for IDUs.

Challenge: Outreach programs for IDUs are needed to promote HIV testing, information dissemination, and education. These programs should also promote condom use and needle exchange.

Prisoners

Status: There are currently no programs for prisoners.

Challenge: Programs should be implemented to promote HIV testing, distribute condoms, and provide health education.

NGO Priorities

Challenge: NGO programs should prioritize MSM, CSWs, and IDUs.

Access to Condoms

Challenges:
- Marketing strategies should be implemented to increase the availability of condoms in key areas (e.g., areas frequented by MSM and CSWs, schools).

- Condom quality control is also needed.

Care Issues and Challenges

Diagnosis

Status: Sixty percent of patients diagnosed with HIV present at advanced stages of infection.

Challenges:
- Anonymous diagnosis centers should be established.

- Testing should be promoted in high-risk populations.

Follow-up Testing

Status: The laboratory network providing CD4 and viral load counts is small, yet over 80 percent of patients had had a CD4 and viral load count.

Challenge: The current laboratory network should be evaluated and strengthened to increase the number of laboratories providing CD4 and viral load tests.

Treatment

Status: Less than half of patients receive antiretroviral treatment; about 30 percent of patients do not receive antiretrovirals because of lack of financial resources.

Challenge: Increase the percentage of patients receiving the treatment they need.

Social Services

Status: Social services provision is limited.

Challenge: Support programs should be implemented for PLWHA, in collaboration with social and labor ministries, through NGOs.

Epidemiological Surveillance Issues and Challenges

Case Definitions, Notification Circuits, and Procedures

Status: Case definitions, notification circuits, and procedures are not defined in working protocols; thus, evaluation and corrective measures are highly labor intensive.

Challenge: National protocols for HIV and AIDS registries are needed specifying the procedures, functions, and responsibilities at each level within the surveillance system. Protocols should also include plans for periodic evaluations of the system.

Underreporting

Status: No data are available, but underreporting is estimated to be high.

Challenge: HIV/AIDS case notification systems should be more exhaustive, and systems for active surveillance are needed.

Protection of Privacy

Status: Current legislation for protection of personal information is not extensive enough to truly guarantee confidentiality of information throughout the diagnosis and treatment process.

Challenge: Better norms are needed to ensure confidentiality of personal information.

Sentinel Surveillance

Status: Sentinel surveillance is deficient in coverage of populations (especially high-risk populations) and in procedure.

Challenge: A plan is needed for sentinel surveillance of HIV and risk factor behavior, specifying populations to monitor, methods, evaluation system, and relationship to decision making in terms of prevention activities. High-risk populations should always be prioritized.

Training

Status: Training in epidemiological surveillance has not been provided at all levels, and there is no integrated plan that consolidates information systems from the general population, sentinel sites, and other sources of information on HIV/AIDS cases.

Challenges:
- An integrated information plan is needed to monitor the epidemic through the national program and multisectorial collaborations.

- Training should be provided to all personnel responsible for epidemiological surveillance, monitoring of interventions, and multisectorial evaluation.

Blood Safety Issues and Challenges

Status: Altruistic, voluntary, and nonremunerated donations are currently combined with other forms of blood donation.

Challenge: Policies are needed to establish altruistic, voluntary, and nonremunerated donations as the only option for donation or transfusion.

Colombia

HIV/AIDS Epidemic Status: Concentrated

Key HIV/AIDS Estimates

- The infection rate is greater than 5 percent in at least one high-risk group.

- Of the adult population, 0.45 percent were estimated to be living with HIV/AIDS at the end of 1999.

- A total of 120,356 people were estimated to be living with HIV/AIDS at the end of 1999.

- An estimated 1,423 people died from HIV/AIDS in 1999.

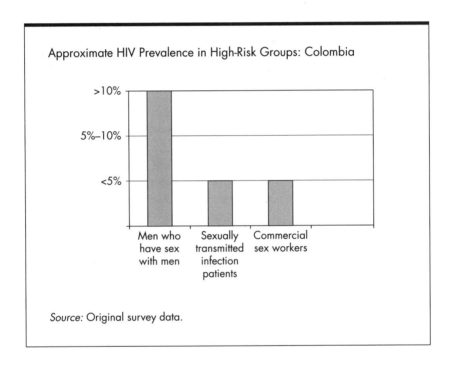

Approximate HIV Prevalence in High-Risk Groups: Colombia

Source: Original survey data.

Important Points about HIV/AIDS in Colombia

- HIV prevalence among teen CSWs has been reported at more than 10 percent.

- Sex between men is the predominant mode of transmission in the highlands, while heterosexual transmission is more common along the Atlantic Coast.

- HIV prevalence in pregnant women is 0.1–0.7 percent.

- HIV prevalence in blood donors is less than 1 percent.

- The major mode of transmission is sex between men.

Funding Resources

The national program does not receive support from international agencies, but it does finance NGOs.

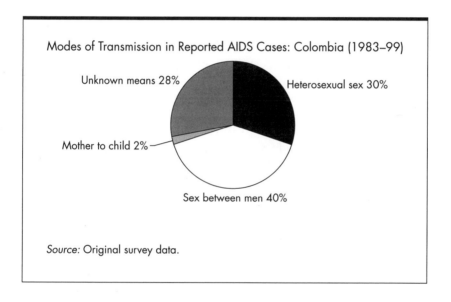

Modes of Transmission in Reported AIDS Cases: Colombia (1983–99)

Unknown means 28%

Heterosexual sex 30%

Mother to child 2%

Sex between men 40%

Source: Original survey data.

Prevention Issues and Challenges

General Population

Status: Some campaigns are under way.

Challenge: Campaigns for the general population should be intensified and should be based on fighting discrimination and promoting condom use.

Adolescents

Status: There is no sexual education or HIV/AIDS education program in the current school curriculum, nor are there interventions for high-risk adolescents.

Challenge: In collaboration with the ministry of health, programs should be designed to incorporate sexual education and HIV/AIDS education in schools. These programs should be carried out in collaboration with youth organizations and NGOs focused on high-risk adolescents.

MSM

Status: Programs have only recently started and require greater strengthening and expansion.

Challenge: Programs should be developed, in collaboration with NGOs and members of the gay movement, focusing on promotion of HIV testing, health education, and condom use promotion.

CSWs

Status: Some programs are under way.

Challenge: Programs should be expanded in large cities to increase access to HIV testing, improve diagnosis and treatment of STIs, and promote systematic condom use.

IDUs

Status: Substantial numbers of intravenous cocaine and heroin users have been found in Colombia.

Challenge: Outreach programs are needed to reach IDUs and promote HIV testing, needle exchange, and condom use.

Prisoners

Status: There are no programs for prisoners.

Challenge: Extensive programs should be implemented that promote HIV testing, distribute condoms, and provide health education.

NGO Priorities

Challenge: The majority of NGO programs should prioritize MSM and IDUs.

Vertical Transmission

Challenge: HIV testing should be offered universally to all pregnant women, and vertical transmission should be reduced through prophylactic antiretroviral treatment.

Care Issues and Challenges

Diagnosis

Status: Fifty percent of patients diagnosed with HIV present at advanced stages of HIV infection or with full-blown AIDS.

Challenge: Anonymous diagnosis centers should be promoted, and HIV testing should be made more available in STI treatment centers.

Treatment

Status: The level of antiretroviral treatment coverage is low.

Psychological and Social Support and Workplace Integration

Status: Psychological and social support and workplace integration activities are limited.

Challenge: In collaboration with self-supported NGOs and social and labor ministries, programs should be organized that respond to these needs.

Epidemiological Surveillance Issues and Challenges

Case Definitions, Notification Circuits, and Procedures

Status: Case definitions, notification circuits, and procedures are not defined in working protocols; thus, evaluation and corrective measures are highly labor intensive.

Challenge: National protocols for HIV and AIDS registries are needed specifying the procedures, functions, and responsibilities at each level within the surveillance system. Protocols should also include plans for periodic evaluations of the system.

Underreporting

Status: Underreporting is estimated at about 80 percent.

Challenge: HIV/AIDS case notification systems should be more exhaustive, and systems for active surveillance are needed.

Protection of Privacy

Status: Current legislation for protection of personal information is not extensive enough to truly guarantee confidentiality of information throughout the diagnosis and treatment process.

Challenge: Better norms are needed to ensure confidentiality of personal information.

Sentinel Surveillance

Status: Sentinel surveillance is deficient in coverage of populations (especially high-risk populations) and in procedure.

Challenge: A plan is needed for sentinel surveillance of HIV and risk factor behavior, specifying populations to monitor, methods, evaluation system, and relationship to decision making in terms of prevention activities. High-risk populations should always be prioritized.

Training

Status: Training in epidemiological surveillance has not been provided at all levels, and there is no integrated plan that consolidates information systems from the general population, sentinel sites, and other sources of information on HIV/AIDS cases.

Challenges:
- An integrated information plan is needed to monitor the epidemic through the national program and multisectorial collaborations.

- Training should be provided to all personnel responsible for epidemiological surveillance, monitoring of interventions, and multisectorial evaluation.

HIV/AIDS Registry

Status: There has been increased access to antiretroviral treatment and a reduction in AIDS cases and mortality.

Challenge: Create a universal registry of HIV infection.

Blood Safety Issues and Challenges

Status: Altruistic, voluntary, and nonremunerated donations are currently combined with other forms of blood donation, and less than 100 percent of the blood supply is tested.

Challenges:
- Policies are needed to establish altruistic, voluntary, and nonremunerated donations as the only option for donation or transfusion.

- Blood testing should be increased, and the blood bank network needs to be strengthened.

Ecuador

HIV/AIDS Epidemic Status: Low Level

Key HIV/AIDS Estimates

- The infection rate is less than 5 percent in high-risk groups.

- Of the adult population, 0.3 percent were estimated to be living with HIV/AIDS at the end of 1999.

- A total of 19,000 people were estimated to be living with HIV/AIDS at the end of 1999.

- An estimated 1,400 people died from HIV/AIDS in 1999.

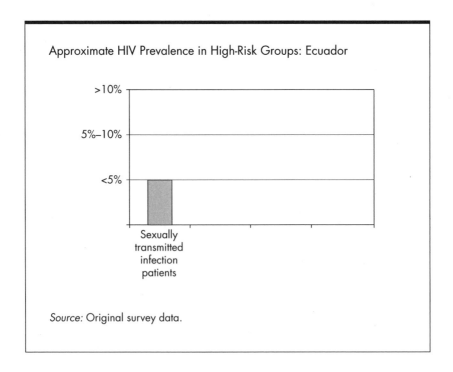

Approximate HIV Prevalence in High-Risk Groups: Ecuador

Source: Original survey data.

Important Points about HIV/AIDS in Ecuador

- Data on HIV/AIDS are scarce.

- Sexually transmitted infections are very prevalent among CSWs and adolescents.

- Condom use and availability are low.

- There is no multisectorial plan for fighting HIV/AIDS. Consensus should be sought among all the relevant players (ministries, professionals, and NGOs).

- HIV prevalence in pregnant women is 0.05 percent (0.3 percent in Guayaquil).

- HIV prevalence is 0.26 percent in blood donors.

Funding Resources

The national HIV/AIDS program receives support from international agencies but does not finance NGOs.

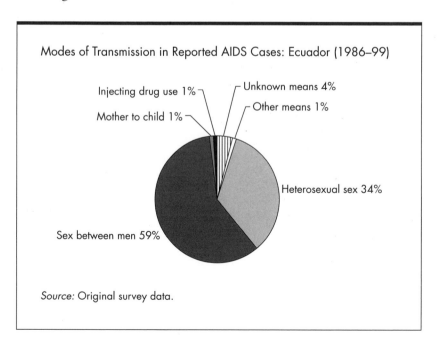

Modes of Transmission in Reported AIDS Cases: Ecuador (1986–99)

Injecting drug use 1%
Mother to child 1%
Unknown means 4%
Other means 1%
Heterosexual sex 34%
Sex between men 59%

Source: Original survey data.

Prevention Issues and Challenges

General Population

Status: Prevention activities have been scarce.

Challenge: Campaigns for the general population (targeting adults and young people) should be planned focused on fighting discrimination and promoting condom use.

Adolescents

Status: There is no sexual education or HIV/AIDS education in schools. The level of schooling up to 14 years of age is very low (only 36 percent).

Challenges:
- In collaboration with the ministry of education, a program should be designed to incorporate HIV/AIDS education in the school curriculum in areas with high prevalence.

- Programs should also be anticipated for high-risk adolescents who do not attend school. These programs could be implemented through NGOs.

MSM

Status: There are no programs for MSM.

Challenges:
- Interventions should be implemented to promote education, prevention, and HIV testing, as well as condom use, in collaboration with NGOs working with the gay movement.

- STI diagnosis centers and centers offering anonymous HIV testing should be expanded and upgraded.

CSWs

Status: There are programs for CSWs, but coverage is limited. There are no programs for male CSWs.

Challenges:

- Programs should be implemented to promote information, prevention, and promotion of HIV testing and condom use in collaboration with NGOs.

- Male and female CSWs should be provided easy access to STI centers for diagnosis and treatment of STIs and HIV testing.

Prisoners

Status: There are no programs for prisoners.

Challenge: Programs should be implemented that promote HIV testing, distribute condoms, and provide information.

Access to Condoms

Status: Access to condoms is limited.

Challenge: Programs are needed to market condoms and increase availability in areas frequented by MSM, young people, and CSWs. Access should also be increased in commercial centers.

Vertical Transmission

Status: HIV testing is not systematically offered to all pregnant women, and the level of coverage with antiretroviral prophylactic treatment is unknown.

Challenge: In collaboration with gynecological associations and health services, HIV testing for pregnant women should be expanded in areas of high prevalence, and antiretroviral prophylactic treatment should be guaranteed for all HIV-positive pregnant women.

Care Issues and Challenges

Diagnosis

Status: Access to HIV testing is limited by cost, discrimination, and lack of demand. Most patients diagnosed with HIV present at advanced stages of HIV infection.

Challenge: Anonymous diagnosis centers should be established in high prevalence areas, where diagnosis would be offered free of charge.

Follow-up Testing

Status: Only 33 percent of patients have had CD4 and viral load counts.

Challenge: The diagnostic laboratory network should be strengthened.

Prophylaxis against Opportunistic Infections

Status: Coverage of diagnosis and treatment of opportunistic infections is low. Over half of patients receive HAART; 36 percent of patients do not receive treatment due to lack of financial resources.

Challenge: Diagnosis and treatment of opportunistic infection should be improved and the percentage of patients receiving the treatment they need increased.

Treatment

Epidemiological Surveillance Issues and Challenges

Case Definitions, Notification Circuits, and Procedures

Status: Case definitions, notification circuits, and procedures are not defined in working protocols; thus, evaluation and corrective measures are highly labor intensive.

Challenge: National protocols for HIV and AIDS registries are needed specifying the procedures, functions, and responsibilities at each level within the surveillance system. Protocols should also include plans for periodic evaluations of the system.

Underreporting

Status: No data are available, but underreporting is estimated to be high.

Challenge: HIV/AIDS case notification systems should be more exhaustive, and systems for active surveillance are needed.

Protection of Privacy

Status: Current legislation for protection of personal information is not extensive enough to truly guarantee confidentiality of information throughout the diagnosis and treatment process.

Challenge: Better norms are needed to ensure confidentiality of personal information.

Sentinel Surveillance

Status: Sentinel surveillance is deficient in coverage of populations (especially high-risk populations) and in procedure.

Challenge: A plan is needed for sentinel surveillance of HIV and risk factor behavior, specifying populations to monitor, methods, evaluation system, and relationship to decision making in terms of prevention activities. High-risk populations should always be prioritized.

Training

Status: Training in epidemiological surveillance has not been provided at all levels, and there is no integrated plan that consolidates information systems from the general population, sentinel sites, and other sources of information on HIV/AIDS cases.

Challenges:
- An integrated information plan is needed to monitor the epidemic through the national program and multisectorial collaborations.

- Training should be provided to all personnel responsible for epidemiological surveillance, monitoring of interventions, and multisectorial evaluation.

Blood Safety Issues and Challenges

Status: Altruistic, voluntary, and nonremunerated donations are currently combined with other forms of blood donation.

Challenge: Policies are needed to establish altruistic, voluntary, and nonremunerated donations as the only option for donation or transfusion.

Peru

HIV/AIDS Epidemic Status: Concentrated

Key HIV/AIDS Estimates

- The infection rate is greater than 5 percent in at least one high-risk group.

- Of the adult population, 0.35 percent were estimated to be living with HIV/AIDS at the end of 1999.

- A total of 48,000 people were estimated to be living with HIV/AIDS at the end of 1999.

- An estimated 4,100 people died from HIV/AIDS in 1999.

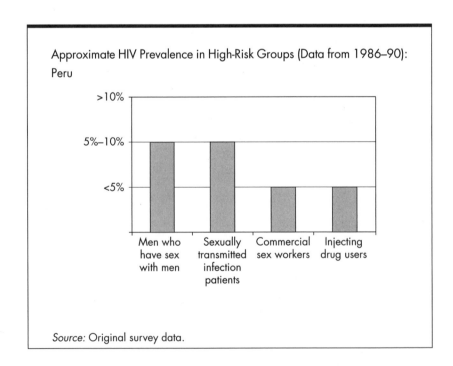

Approximate HIV Prevalence in High-Risk Groups (Data from 1986–90): Peru

Source: Original survey data.

Important Points about HIV/AIDS in Peru

- HIV/AIDS is concentrated among the poor in coastal cities, especially in Lima.

- HIV is increasing in Iquitos as a result of gay tourism.

- STIs are high, but treatment is rarely sought.

- HIV prevalence in pregnant women is less than 1 percent; prevalences of 0.23–0.58 percent have been found in 15- to 24-year-olds in Lima (0.3 percent in 1999).

- HIV prevalence is 0.24 percent in blood donors.

- The most common modes of transmission are sex between men and heterosexual sex.

Funding Resources

The national program receives support from international agencies but does not finance NGOs.

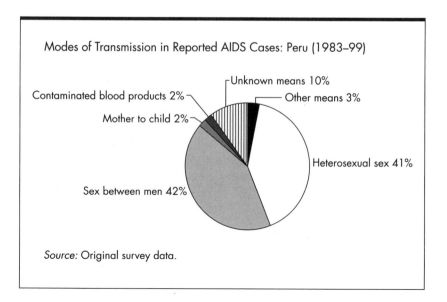

Modes of Transmission in Reported AIDS Cases: Peru (1983–99)

Unknown means 10%
Other means 3%
Contaminated blood products 2%
Mother to child 2%
Heterosexual sex 41%
Sex between men 42%

Source: Original survey data.

Prevention Issues and Challenges

General Population

Status: Campaigns for information and prevention and condom promotion have been scarce.

Challenge: Campaigns for young people and adults should be increased focused on fighting discrimination and promoting condom use.

Adolescents

Status: There are no sexual education or HIV/AIDS education programs in schools.

Challenges:
- In collaboration with the ministry of education, programs should be incorporated into the school curriculum.

- Interventions for high-risk adolescents should be increased.

CSWs

Status: Some programs are under way.

Challenge: Programs should be expanded in large cities to increase access to HIV testing and to increase testing available at STI treatment centers to ensure control and promotion of HIV testing.

Prisoners

Status: Programs have recently been developed but offer limited coverage.

Challenge: Programs should be implemented that provide health education, distribute condoms, and provide HIV testing.

Access to Condoms

Challenges:
- Access to condoms should be increased, especially in areas frequented by MSM and young people.

- Programs for condom quality control should be developed.

NGOs

Status: There are few NGOs working in this country.

Challenge: Collaborative community movements should be facilitated, prioritizing work with CSWs and MSM.

Care Issues and Challenges

Diagnosis

Status: Access to testing is limited by cost and risk of discrimination. Eighty percent of patients diagnosed with HIV present at advanced stages of HIV infection or with full-blown AIDS.

Challenge: Anonymous diagnosis centers should be expanded, and sites providing free diagnosis should be increased.

Follow-up Testing

Status: Only 14 percent of patients have had at least one CD4 and viral load count.

Challenge: The laboratory network providing diagnostic tests must be strengthened.

Treatment

Status: Seventy-two percent of patients do not have access to anti-retroviral treatment because of lack of financial resources, and only 10 percent receive HAART.

Challenge: Programs need to increase the percentage of patients receiving the treatment they need.

Social Support and Workplace Integration

Status: Social support and workplace integration activities are limited.

Challenge: In collaboration with NGOs and social and labor ministries, programs for social and employment support should be organized.

Epidemiological Surveillance Issues and Challenges

Case Definitions, Notification Circuits, and Procedures

Status: Case definitions, notification circuits, and procedures are not defined in working protocols; thus, evaluation and corrective measures are highly labor intensive.

Challenge: National protocols for HIV and AIDS registries are needed specifying the procedures, functions, and responsibilities at each level within the surveillance system. Protocols should also include plans for periodic evaluations of the system.

Underreporting

Status: No data are available, but underreporting is estimated to be moderate to high.

Challenge: HIV/AIDS case notification systems should be more exhaustive, and already existing systems for active surveillance should be expanded.

Protection of Privacy

Status: Current legislation for protection of personal information is not extensive enough to truly guarantee confidentiality of information throughout the diagnosis and treatment process.

Challenge: Better norms are needed to ensure confidentiality of personal information.

Sentinel Surveillance

Status: Sentinel surveillance is deficient in coverage of populations (especially high-risk populations) and in procedure.

Challenge: A plan is needed for sentinel surveillance of HIV and risk factor behavior, specifying populations to monitor, methods, evaluation system, and relationship to decision making in terms of prevention activities. High-risk populations should always be prioritized.

Training

Status: Training in epidemiological surveillance has not been provided at all levels, and there is no integrated plan that consolidates information systems from the general population, sentinel sites, and other sources of information on HIV/AIDS cases.

Challenges:
- An integrated information plan is needed to monitor the epidemic through the national program and multisectorial collaborations.

- Training should be provided to all personnel responsible for epidemiological surveillance, monitoring of interventions, and multisectorial evaluation.

Blood Safety Issues and Challenges

Status: Altruistic, voluntary, and nonremunerated donations are currently combined with other forms of blood donation.

Challenge: Policies are needed to establish altruistic, voluntary, and nonremunerated donations as the only option for donation or transfusion.

Bolivia

HIV/AIDS Epidemic Status: Low Level

Key HIV/AIDS Estimates

- The infection rate is less than 5 percent in high-risk groups.

- Of the adult population, 0.1 percent were estimated to be living with HIV/AIDS at the end of 1999.

- A total of 4,200 people were estimated to be living with HIV/AIDS at the end of 1999.

- An estimated 380 people died from HIV/AIDS in 1999.

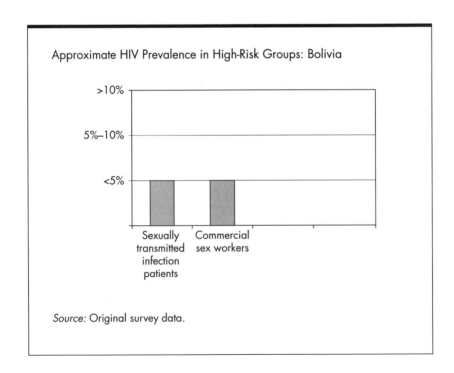

Approximate HIV Prevalence in High-Risk Groups: Bolivia

Source: Original survey data.

Important Points about HIV/AIDS in Bolivia

- HIV/AIDS is concentrated in urban areas of the central corridor: La Paz, Cochabamba, and Santa Cruz.

- STI levels, including syphilis and gonorrhea, are increasing.

- Less than half of donated blood is screened for HIV.

- STIs are high, but treatment is rarely sought.

- HIV prevalence in pregnant women is 0.0–0.5 percent.

- The most common mode of transmission is heterosexual sex.

Funding Resources

The national program does not receive support from international agencies and does not finance NGOs. There is no multisectorial plan for fighting HIV/AIDS.

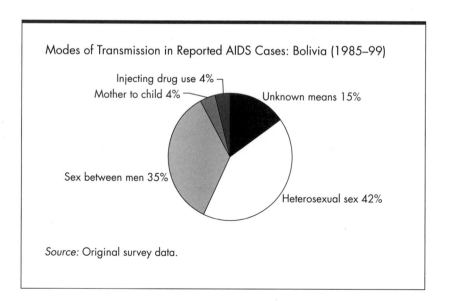

Modes of Transmission in Reported AIDS Cases: Bolivia (1985–99)

Injecting drug use 4%
Mother to child 4%
Unknown means 15%
Sex between men 35%
Heterosexual sex 42%

Source: Original survey data.

Overall Issues and Challenges

- A single case definition is needed for AIDS.

- A system for HIV case notification should be implemented.

- A national protocol should be established for registering HIV and AIDS cases.

- Better norms are needed for protecting the confidentiality of personal information.

- Personnel working in epidemiological surveillance require training, and a national HIV surveillance plan should be developed that includes behavioral risk factor surveillance. Such programs should prioritize high-risk and variable risk groups.

- The exhaustiveness of HIV and AIDS case notification should be increased through implementing more active surveillance systems, at least in large cities.

- Information must be linked to decision making.

- Periodic evaluations of the surveillance system should be planned.

Prevention Issues and Challenges

Status: There are no data available on prevention activities for the general population or specific groups.

Challenges: It is necessary to design and implement a prevention strategy. This strategy should prioritize the following interventions:

- Campaigns for the general population and young people based on fighting discrimination and promoting condom use

- Programs for men who have sex with men, in collaboration with NGOs, in order to inform, provide services for STI diagnosis, and promote HIV testing and condom use

- Programs for commercial sex workers focused on facilitating access to STI diagnostic and treatment services, providing information, and promoting HIV testing and condom use

- Prison programs focused on providing information, promoting HIV testing, and distributing condoms.

Vertical Transmission

Status: HIV testing is not offered to pregnant women.

Challenge: In collaboration with gynecological societies and health services, programs should be implemented to facilitate offering HIV testing to all pregnant women.

Care Issues and Challenges

Diagnosis

Status: Access to testing is limited by cost, risk of discrimination, and lack of demand. Most patients diagnosed with HIV present at advanced stages of infection.

Challenge: Anonymous diagnosis centers should be expanded in areas of high prevalence, and testing should be free.

Follow-up Testing

Status: Only 10 percent of patients have had at least one CD4 and viral load count.

Challenge: The laboratory network providing diagnostic tests must be strengthened.

Diagnosis and Treatment of Opportunistic Infections

Status: Coverage is low, and use of antiretroviral treatment is inconsistent with current standards.

Challenge: Programs for continuous training of clinicians in the management and treatment of HIV/AIDS patients and associated infections are needed.

Epidemiological Surveillance Issues and Challenges

Case Definitions, Notification Circuits, and Procedures

Status: Case definitions, notification circuits, and procedures are not defined in working protocols; thus, evaluation and corrective measures are highly labor intensive.

Challenge: National protocols for HIV and AIDS registries are needed specifying the procedures, functions, and responsibilities at each level within the surveillance system. Protocols should also include plans for periodic evaluations of the system.

Underreporting

Status: Underreporting is estimated at about 30 percent for HIV and 60 percent for AIDS.

Challenge: HIV/AIDS case notification systems should be more exhaustive, and active surveillance systems should be facilitated.

Protection of Privacy

Status: Current legislation for protection of personal information is not extensive enough to truly guarantee confidentiality of information throughout the diagnosis and treatment process.

Challenge: Better norms are needed to ensure confidentiality of personal information.

Sentinel Surveillance

Status: Sentinel surveillance is deficient in coverage of populations (especially high-risk populations) and in procedure.

Challenge: A plan is needed for sentinel surveillance of HIV and risk factor behavior, specifying populations to monitor, methods, evaluation system, and relationship to decision making in terms of prevention activities. High-risk populations should always be prioritized.

Training

Status: Training in epidemiological surveillance has not been provided at all levels, and there is no integrated plan that consolidates information systems from the general population, sentinel sites, and other sources of information on HIV/AIDS cases.

Challenges:
- An integrated information plan is needed to monitor the epidemic through the national program and multisectorial collaborations.

- Training should be provided to all personnel responsible for epidemiological surveillance, monitoring of interventions, and multisectorial evaluation.

Blood Safety Issues and Challenges

Status: Altruistic, voluntary, and nonremunerated donations are currently combined with other forms of blood donation. Only 40 percent of blood donations are tested for HIV.

Challenges:
- Policies are needed to establish altruistic, voluntary, and nonremunerated donations as the only option for donation or transfusion.

- The percentage of blood tested for HIV must increase through strengthening infrastructure and training in blood banks.

Argentina

HIV/AIDS Epidemic Status: Concentrated

Key HIV/AIDS Estimates

- The infection rate is greater than 5 percent in at least one high-risk group.

- Of the adult population, 0.66 percent were estimated to be living with HIV/AIDS at the end of 1999.

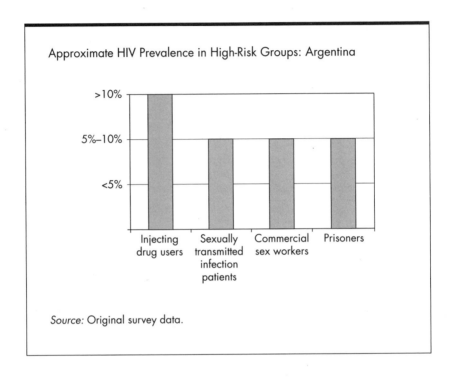

Approximate HIV Prevalence in High-Risk Groups: Argentina

Source: Original survey data.

- A total of 130,000 people were estimated to be living with HIV/AIDS at the end of 1999.
- An estimated 1,800 people died from HIV/AIDS in 1999.

Important Points about HIV/AIDS in Argentina

- HIV prevalence in pregnant women is 0.56–0.66 percent (as high as 2 percent in urban areas).
- HIV prevalence is 0.13 percent in blood donors.
- The most common mode of transmission is injecting drug use.

Funding Resources

The national HIV/AIDS program receives support from international agencies and finances NGOs. The national program budget is one of the highest in the Southern Cone.

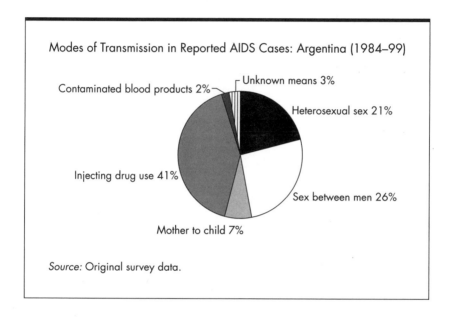

Modes of Transmission in Reported AIDS Cases: Argentina (1984–99)

Contaminated blood products 2%

Unknown means 3%

Heterosexual sex 21%

Injecting drug use 41%

Sex between men 26%

Mother to child 7%

Source: Original survey data.

Prevention Issues and Challenges

General Population

Status: There have been few campaigns for the general population; none has focused on condom promotion.

Challenge: Campaigns fighting discrimination and promoting condom use should be developed.

Adolescents

Status: There is no plan in the ministry of health for including sexual education or AIDS education in the school curriculums.

Challenge: In collaboration with the ministry of health, sexual education, AIDS education, and drug education programs should be initiated in schools, beginning in the areas with highest HIV prevalence.

IDUs

Status: Harm reduction programs have only recently begun, and their coverage is insufficient.

Challenge: Urgently needed activities include needle exchange programs, condom use, HIV testing promotion (via NGOs), and establishment of centers for health care and services for drug addicts.

Prisoners

Status: Prison programs are scarce and need to be expanded.

Challenges:
• These programs should be expanded to cover more prisoners and should include promotion of condom use and HIV testing, along with health education.

• Harm reduction programs should be planned focused on needle exchange and instruction on how to clean instruments. These programs should target the prisons with the highest prevalence of IDUs.

NGO Priorities

Challenge: The majority of NGO programs should prioritize MSM and IDUs.

Vertical Transmission

Status: HIV testing is offered to about 70 percent of pregnant women, and 90 percent of HIV-positive pregnant women are offered antiretroviral therapy as a prophylactic measure.

Challenge: HIV testing should be offered to all pregnant women, and antiretroviral prophylaxis should be given to all HIV-positive pregnant women.

Care Issues and Challenges

Diagnosis

Status: Access to HIV testing is limited. Sixty percent of patients diagnosed with HIV present at advanced stages of infection.

Challenge: Anonymous diagnosis centers should be established in areas with the highest prevalence.

Follow-up Testing

Status: Eighty percent of HIV/AIDS patients have had a CD4 and viral load count.

Challenge: The laboratory network should be strengthened and expanded to provide greater coverage of diagnostic and monitoring tests.

Prophylaxis against Opportunistic Infections

Status: Coverage is limited (55 percent).

Challenge: Programs for continuous training of clinicians in the management and treatment of HIV/AIDS patients and associated infections are needed.

Psychological and Social Support and Workplace Integration

Status: Psychological and social support and workplace integration activities are limited.

Challenge: In collaboration with self-supported NGOs and social and labor ministries, programs should be organized that respond to these needs.

Epidemiological Surveillance Issues and Challenges

Case Definitions, Notification Circuits, and Procedures

Status: Case definitions, notification circuits, and procedures are not defined in working protocols; thus, evaluation and corrective measures are highly labor intensive.

Challenge: National protocols for HIV and AIDS registries are needed specifying the procedures, functions, and responsibilities at each level within the surveillance system. Protocols should also include plans for periodic evaluations of the system.

Underreporting

Status: Underreporting is estimated at 20 percent.

Challenge: HIV/AIDS case notification systems should be more exhaustive, and active surveillance systems are needed.

Protection of Privacy

Status: Current legislation for protection of personal information is not extensive enough to truly guarantee confidentiality of information throughout the diagnosis and treatment process.

Challenge: Better norms are needed to ensure confidentiality of personal information.

Sentinel Surveillance

Status: Sentinel surveillance is deficient in coverage of populations (especially high-risk populations) and in procedure.

Challenge: A plan is needed for sentinel surveillance of HIV and risk factor behavior, specifying populations to monitor, methods, evaluation system, and relationship to decision making in terms of prevention activities. High-risk populations should always be prioritized.

Training

Status: Training in epidemiological surveillance has not been provided at all levels, and there is no integrated plan that consolidates information systems from the general population, sentinel sites, and other sources of information on HIV/AIDS cases.

Challenges:
- An integrated information plan is needed to monitor the epidemic through the national program and multisectorial collaborations.

- Training should be provided to all personnel responsible for epidemiological surveillance, monitoring of interventions, and multisectorial evaluation.

HIV/AIDS Registry

Status: There has been increased access to antiretroviral treatment and a reduction in AIDS cases and mortality.

Challenge: A universal registry of HIV infection should be created.

Blood Safety Issues and Challenges

Status: Altruistic, voluntary, and nonremunerated donations are currently combined with other forms of blood donation. Ninety-five percent of the blood supply is tested.

Challenges:
- Policies are needed to establish altruistic, voluntary, and nonremunerated donations as the only option for donation or transfusion.

- Blood testing should cover 100 percent of donated blood. This would be possible through improving and expanding the infrastructure of blood banks.

Paraguay

HIV/AIDS Epidemic Status: Concentrated

Key HIV/AIDS Estimates

- Overall, data from Paraguay are scarce.

- The infection rate is less than 5 percent in high-risk groups.

- Of the adult population, 0.11 percent were estimated to be living with HIV/AIDS at the end of 1999.

- A total of 3,000 people were estimated to be living with HIV/AIDS at the end of 1999.

- An estimated 220 people died from HIV/AIDS in 1999.

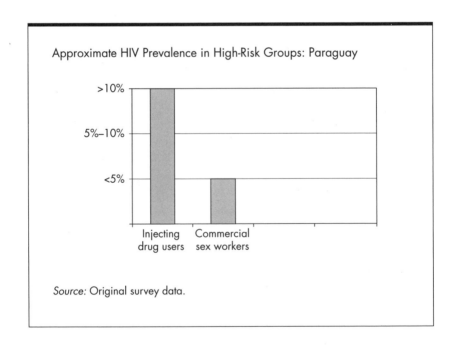

Approximate HIV Prevalence in High-Risk Groups: Paraguay

Source: Original survey data.

Important Points about HIV/AIDS in Paraguay

- HIV prevalence in pregnant women is less than 0.1 percent.

- The estimated prevalence among military recruits is 1 percent.

- HIV prevalence in blood donors is 0.17 percent.

- The most common modes of transmission are heterosexual sex and sex between men.

Funding Resources

The national program receives support from international agencies but does not finance NGOs. The national program budget is one of the highest in the Southern Cone.

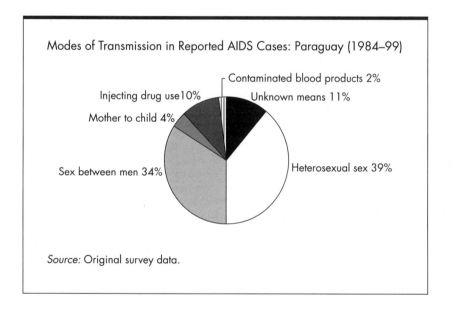

Modes of Transmission in Reported AIDS Cases: Paraguay (1984–99)

Contaminated blood products 2%

Injecting drug use 10%

Unknown means 11%

Mother to child 4%

Sex between men 34%

Heterosexual sex 39%

Source: Original survey data.

Overall Issues and Challenges

Status: The level of multisectorial agreement in the national program is low. There is little coherence in government or NGOs in the fight against HIV/AIDS. There is no national commission for the evaluation of the national HIV/AIDS program.

Challenge: More multisectorial collaboration needs to be established and links built between the government and NGOs. A national commission for evaluating the national HIV/AIDS program should be established.

Prevention Issues and Challenges

MSM

Status: Programs have recently begun and require more strengthening and expansion.

Challenge: In collaboration with NGOs and the gay movement, programs should focus on promotion of HIV testing, health education, and condom use promotion.

CSWs

Status: Some programs are under way.

Challenge: It is necessary to expand programs for CSWs in large cities. These programs should help increase access to HIV testing, distribute condoms, and improve access and services at health centers and STI treatment centers.

IDUs

Status: Programs for IDUs are insufficient.

Challenge: Programs are needed for needle exchange, promotion of HIV testing, and condom use. Such activities could be carried out by NGOs, health care centers, and centers for drug addicts.

Prisoners

Status: Prison programs are scarce and require expansion.

Challenges:
- These programs should be expanded to cover more prisoners and should include promotion of condom use and HIV testing, along with health education.

- Harm reduction programs should be planned focused on needle exchange and instruction on how to clean instruments. These programs should target the prisons with the highest prevalence of IDUs.

NGO Priorities

Challenge: NGO programs and projects should prioritize MSM.

Vertical Transmission

Status: It is unknown how many pregnant women are offered HIV testing or antiretroviral prophylaxis.

Challenge: Programs should be implemented that evaluate the rate of HIV testing and actual cases in this population.

Care Issues and Challenges

Diagnosis

Status: More than half of patients are diagnosed at the stage of AIDS or advanced HIV infection. The main barriers to testing are the lack of demand, social discrimination, and low availability of diagnosis centers.

Challenge: Anonymous HIV diagnosis centers are needed, and the test should be available at STI treatment centers.

Follow-up Testing

Status: Only 55 percent of HIV/AIDS patients have had a CD4 and viral load count.

Challenge: The laboratory network should be evaluated and strengthened to increase the number of laboratories providing diagnostic and monitoring tests.

Treatment

Status: One out of every four patients does not receive antiretroviral therapy because of lack of financial resources. Forty-four percent of patients receive HAART.

Challenge: Improve the percentage of patients receiving the treatment they need.

Psychological and Social Support and Workplace Integration

Status: Psychological and social support and workplace integration activities are limited.

Challenge: Self-supported community movements and social protection programs for people living with HIV/AIDS should be supported in collaboration with social and labor ministries.

Epidemiological Surveillance Issues and Challenges

Case Definitions, Notification Circuits, and Procedures

Status: Case definitions, notification circuits, and procedures are not defined in working protocols; thus, evaluation and corrective measures are highly labor intensive.

Challenge: National protocols for HIV and AIDS registries are needed specifying the procedures, functions, and responsibilities at each level within the surveillance system. Protocols should also include plans for periodic evaluations of the system.

Underreporting

Status: No data are available, but underreporting is estimated to be moderate to high.

Challenge: HIV/AIDS case notification systems should be more exhaustive, and systems for active surveillance are needed.

Protection of Privacy

Status: Current legislation for protection of personal information is not extensive enough to truly guarantee confidentiality of information throughout the diagnosis and treatment process.

Challenge: Better norms are needed to ensure confidentiality of personal information.

Sentinel Surveillance

Status: Sentinel surveillance is deficient in coverage of populations (especially high-risk populations) and in procedure.

Challenge: A plan is needed for sentinel surveillance of HIV and risk factor behavior, specifying populations to monitor, methods, evaluation system, and relationship to decision making in terms of prevention activities. High-risk populations should always be prioritized.

Training

Status: Training in epidemiological surveillance has not been provided at all levels, and there is no integrated plan that consolidates information systems from the general population, sentinel sites, and other sources of information on HIV/AIDS cases.

Challenges:
- An integrated information plan is needed to monitor the epidemic through the national program and multisectorial collaborations.

- Training should be provided to all personnel responsible for epidemiological surveillance, monitoring of interventions, and multisectorial evaluation.

Blood Safety Issues and Challenges

Status: Altruistic, voluntary, and nonremunerated donations are currently combined with other forms of blood donation.

Challenge: Policies are needed to establish altruistic, voluntary, and non-remunerated donations as the only option for donation or transfusion.

Uruguay

HIV/AIDS Epidemic Status: Concentrated

Key HIV/AIDS Estimates

- The infection rate is greater than 5 percent in at least one high-risk group.

- Of the adult population, 0.37 percent were estimated to be living with HIV/AIDS at the end of 1999.

- A total of 6,000 people were estimated to be living with HIV/AIDS at the end of 1999.

- An estimated 150 people died from HIV/AIDS in 1999.

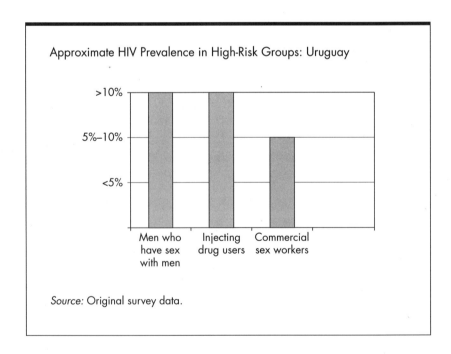

Approximate HIV Prevalence in High-Risk Groups: Uruguay

Source: Original survey data.

Important Points about HIV/AIDS in Uruguay

- HIV prevalence in pregnant women is 0.23 percent.

- In 1993, 6 percent of military recruits were HIV infected.

- HIV prevalence in blood donors is 0.6 percent.

- The most common mode of transmission is sex between men.

Funding Resources

The national HIV/AIDS program receives support from international agencies and finances NGOs.

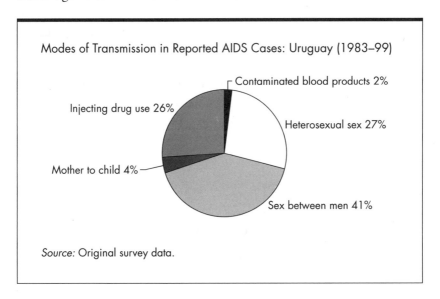

Modes of Transmission in Reported AIDS Cases: Uruguay (1983–99)

Contaminated blood products 2%

Injecting drug use 26%

Heterosexual sex 27%

Mother to child 4%

Sex between men 41%

Source: Original survey data.

Prevention Issues and Challenges

Adolescents

Status: Coverage of sexual education and HIV/AIDS education is less than 50 percent in public schools.

Challenges:
- Coverage of school-based education programs should expand, especially in the cities that are most affected.

- Programs for high-risk adolescents and young people who do not attend school should also be expanded.

MSM

Status: There are some occasional activities that only recently started and have limited coverage.

Challenge: Programs should be developed, in collaboration with NGOs and members of the gay movement, focusing on promotion of HIV testing, health education, and promotion of condom use.

CSWs

Status: Some programs are under way.

Challenge: It is necessary to expand programs for CSWs in large cities. These programs should help promote HIV testing, distribute condoms to all CSWs, and improve access and testing in health care centers and STI treatment centers.

IDUs

Status: The level of HIV infection in IDUs is high, yet there are still no harm reduction programs in place.

Challenge: Programs are needed for needle exchange, promotion of HIV testing and condom use, information dissemination, and health education, as well as testing in drug addiction clinics. Such activities could be carried out by NGOs, health care centers, and centers for drug addicts.

Prisoners

Status: Prison programs are scarce and require expansion.

Challenges:
- These programs should be expanded to cover more prisoners and should include promotion of condom use and HIV testing, along with health education.

- Harm reduction programs should be planned focused on needle exchange and instruction on how to clean instruments. These programs should target the prisons with the highest prevalence of IDUs.

NGO Priorities

Challenge: In terms of financing, NGOs should prioritize IDU-based programs.

Care Issues and Challenges

Diagnosis

Status: Access to HIV testing is limited by discrimination and lack of demand. Sixty percent of patients are diagnosed in advanced stages of infection.

Challenge: Anonymous HIV diagnosis centers are needed in areas of high prevalence.

Treatment

Status: Fifty-five percent of HIV/AIDS patients are receiving HAART; 8 percent do not take HAART because of lack of financial resources.

Challenge: Programs are needed to increase the percentage of patients who receive the treatment they need.

Psychological and Social Support and Workplace Integration

Status: Psychological and social support and workplace integration activities are limited.

Challenge: In collaboration with NGOs and social and labor ministries, programs for improving social and psychological services should be organized.

Epidemiological Surveillance Issues and Challenges

Case Definitions, Notification Circuits, and Procedures

Status: Case definitions, notification circuits, and procedures are not defined in working protocols; thus, evaluation and corrective measures are highly labor intensive.

Challenge: National protocols for HIV and AIDS registries are needed specifying the procedures, functions, and responsibilities at each level within the surveillance system. Protocols should also include plans for periodic evaluations of the system.

Underreporting

Status: Underreporting is estimated at 10–15 percent.

Challenge: HIV/AIDS case notification systems should be more exhaustive, and already existing systems for active surveillance should be expanded.

Protection of Privacy

Status: Current legislation for protection of personal information is not extensive enough to truly guarantee confidentiality of information throughout the diagnosis and treatment process.

Challenge: Better norms are needed to ensure confidentiality of personal information.

Sentinel Surveillance

Status: Sentinel surveillance is deficient in coverage of populations (especially high-risk populations) and in procedure.

Challenge: A plan is needed for sentinel surveillance of HIV and risk factor behavior, specifying populations to monitor, methods, evaluation system, and relationship to decision making in terms of prevention activities. High-risk populations should always be prioritized.

Training

Status: Training in epidemiological surveillance has not been provided at all levels, and there is no integrated plan that consolidates information systems from the general population, sentinel sites, and other sources of information on HIV/AIDS cases.

Challenges:
- An integrated information plan is needed to monitor the epidemic through the national program and multisectorial collaborations.

- Training should be provided to all personnel responsible for epidemiological surveillance, monitoring of interventions, and multisectorial evaluation.

Blood Safety Issues and Challenges

Status: Altruistic, voluntary, and nonremunerated donations are currently combined with other forms of blood donation.

Challenge: Policies are needed to establish altruistic, voluntary, and nonremunerated donations as the only option for donation or transfusion.

Chile

HIV/AIDS Epidemic Status: Concentrated

Key HIV/AIDS Estimates

- The infection rate is less than 5 percent in high-risk groups.

- Of the adult population, 0.19 percent were estimated to be living with HIV/AIDS at the end of 1999.

- A total of 15,000 people were estimated to be living with HIV/AIDS at the end of 1999.

- An estimated 1,000 people died from HIV/AIDS in 1999.

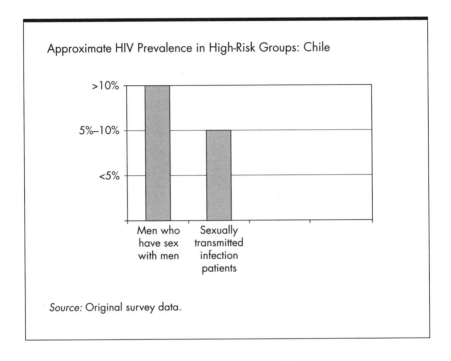

Approximate HIV Prevalence in High-Risk Groups: Chile

Source: Original survey data.

Important Points about HIV/AIDS in Chile

- HIV prevalence in pregnant women is 0.1 percent.
- Heterosexual transmission of HIV is increasing, although sex between men still accounts for most cases.
- HIV prevalence in blood donors is less than 0.1 percent.
- The most common mode of transmission is sex between men.

Funding Resources

The national HIV/AIDS program receives support from international agencies and finances nongovernmental organizations (NGOs). The national program budget is one of the highest in the Southern Cone.

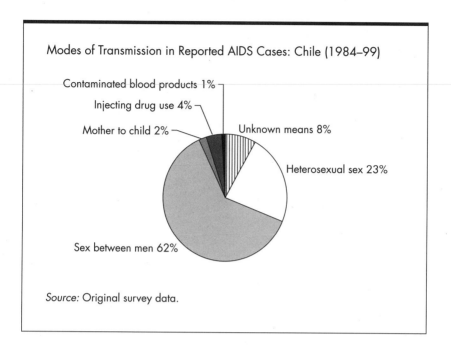

Modes of Transmission in Reported AIDS Cases: Chile (1984–99)

Contaminated blood products 1%
Injecting drug use 4%
Mother to child 2%
Unknown means 8%
Heterosexual sex 23%
Sex between men 62%

Source: Original survey data.

Prevention Issues and Challenges

General Population

Status: There have been few information and communication campaigns, and none of the campaigns thus far have promoted condom use.

Challenge: Campaigns fighting discrimination and promoting condom use should be developed and implemented.

Adolescents

Status: There is currently no plan within the ministry of education for including sexual education, including HIV/AIDS education, in the school curriculum.

Challenges:
• Beginning in areas with high HIV prevalence, sexual education, HIV/AIDS education, and drug education should be introduced

into the school curriculums in collaboration with national education authorities.

- With the collaboration of NGOs and youth associations, programs targeting high-risk adolescents should be established.

MSM

Status: There are some occasional activities that only recently started and have limited coverage.

Challenge: Programs should be developed, in collaboration with NGOs and members of the gay movement, focusing on promotion of HIV testing, health education, and promotion of condom use.

CSWs

Status: Some programs are under way.

Challenge: It is necessary to expand programs for CSWs in large cities and to develop programs for male CSWs. These programs should help increase access to HIV testing, diagnosis and treatment of STIs, and systematic condom use.

IDUs

Status: Harm reduction programs have recently begun, and their scope is limited.

Challenge: Programs are needed for needle exchange and promotion of HIV testing and condom use. Such activities could be carried out by NGOs, health care centers, and centers for drug addicts.

Prisoners

Status: Prison programs are scarce and require expansion.

Challenges:
- These programs should be expanded to cover more prisoners and should include promotion of condom use and HIV testing, along with health education.

- Harm reduction programs should be focused on needle exchange and instruction on how to clean instruments. These programs should target the prisons with the highest prevalence of IDUs.

Vertical Transmission

Status: It is unknown how many pregnant women are offered the HIV test, but antiretroviral prophylaxis is offered to 100 percent of HIV-positive pregnant women.

Challenge: The HIV test should be offered to all pregnant women, and antiretroviral prophylaxis should be given to all HIV-positive pregnant women.

Care Issues and Challenges

Diagnosis

Status: Access to HIV testing could improve. The main barriers to testing are the cost and social discrimination.

Challenge: Anonymous HIV diagnosis centers are needed, and testing should be promoted in high-risk groups.

Follow-up Testing

Status: Seventy-two percent of HIV/AIDS patients have had a CD4 and viral load count.

Challenge: The laboratory network should be strengthened and expanded to provide greater coverage of diagnostic and monitoring tests.

Psychological and Social Support and Workplace Integration

Status: Psychological and social support and workplace integration activities are limited.

Challenge: In collaboration with self-supported NGOs and social and labor ministries, programs should be organized that respond to these needs.

Epidemiological Surveillance Issues and Challenges

Case Definitions, Notification Circuits, and Procedures

Status: Case definitions, notification circuits, and procedures are not defined in working protocols; thus, evaluation and corrective measures are highly labor intensive.

Challenge: National protocols for HIV and AIDS registries are needed specifying the procedures, functions, and responsibilities at each level within the surveillance system. Protocols should also include plans for periodic evaluations of the system.

Underreporting

Status: Underreporting is estimated at 14 percent.

Challenge: HIV/AIDS case notification systems should be more exhaustive, and active surveillance systems are needed.

Protection of Privacy

Status: Current legislation for protection of personal information is not extensive enough to truly guarantee confidentiality of information throughout the diagnosis and treatment process.

Challenge: Better norms are needed to ensure confidentiality of personal information.

Sentinel Surveillance

Status: Sentinel surveillance is deficient in coverage of populations (especially high-risk populations) and in procedure.

Challenge: A plan is needed for sentinel surveillance of HIV and risk factor behavior, specifying populations to monitor, methods, evaluation system, and relationship to decision making in terms of prevention activities. High-risk populations should always be prioritized.

Training

Status: Training in epidemiological surveillance has not been provided at all levels, and there is no integrated plan that consolidates information systems from the general population, sentinel sites, and other sources of information on HIV/AIDS cases.

Challenges:

- An integrated information plan is needed to monitor the epidemic through the national program and multisectorial collaborations.

- Training should be provided to all personnel responsible for epidemiological surveillance, monitoring of interventions, and multisectorial evaluation.

HIV/AIDS Registry

Status: There has been increased access to antiretroviral treatment and a reduction in AIDS cases and mortality.

Challenge: A universal registry of HIV infection should be created.

Blood Safety Issues and Challenges

Status: Altruistic, voluntary, and nonremunerated donations are currently combined with other forms of blood donation.

Challenge: Policies are needed to establish altruistic, voluntary, and nonremunerated donations as the only option for donation or transfusion.

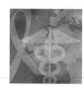

Collaborators in the Study

National Program Directors

Mabel Bianco—Argentina
Vito Rivas Vargas—Bolivia
Paulo Teixeira—Brazil
Anabela Arredondo-Paz and Edith Ortiz Núñez—Chile
Carlos Hernández—Colombia
Ignacio Salom-Echeverría—Costa Rica
María Helena Acosta—Ecuador
Gladys de Bonilla—El Salvador
Dori Lucas-Alecio—Guatemala
Marco Alvarenga—Honduras
Patricia Uribe-Zúñiga—Mexico
Matilde Román Rivas—Nicaragua
Norma García Paredes—Panama
Nicolás Aguayo—Paraguay
Lourdes Kunsunoki—Peru
Margarita Serra—Uruguay
Deisy Matos—Venezuela

Nongovernmental Organizations

Argentina

Silvia Kurlat—Federación Argentina de SIDA y Salud (FASS)
Gustavo Karaman—Asociación Civil Don Jaime de Nevares
Rafael Fedra—Sigla
Graciela Touzé and Diana Rossi—Intercambios
Carlos Mendes—NEXO

Bolivia

Jayne Lyons—Care, Bolivia
Edgar Valdéz Carrizo—Instituto de Desarrollo Humano (IDH)
Edwing Holguín—CAIASIDA (Centro Integral del Adolescente y
    SIDA)
Violeta Ross—Mas Vida (Asociación Seropositivos)
Liesolotte de Barragán—Fundación San Gabriel

Brazil

Rosa Beatriz Marinho—GAPA/BA
Veriano Terto Jr.—ABIA
Célia Ruthes—GAPA/RS
J. Humberto Mello—RNP+ (Núcleo de São José do Rio Preto)
Eduardo Luis Barbosa—GIV/SP

Chile

Daniel Esteban Palma Sepúlveda—FRENASIDA
Herminda González—Fundación Margen
Bernardina Flores Rivas and Marco Becerra Silva—Corporación
    Chilena de Prevención del SIDA

Colombia

Jennypher Calderón and Alfredo Mejía—Liga Colombiana de
    Lucha contra el SIDA

Constanza Molina—Eco de Libertad
Sulma Manco—CORMUJER
Fabián Medina—Fundación Darse

Costa Rica

Miriam Fernández Esquivel—Fundesida
María Solano—Asociación Costarricense de Personas que Viven
con VIH/SIDA
Cristina Garita—Fundación VIDA
Edgar Mora González—Fundación Niños de Dios
Daria Suárez—CIPAC/DDHH

Ecuador

Orlando Montoya Herrera—Fundación Ecuatoriana Equidad
Ana Cordero Cueva—Fundación Pájara Pinta
Irene León—FEDAEPS
Margarita Quevedo—Kimirina
María Cecilia Gutiérrez—Fundación Dios, Vida y Esperanza

El Salvador

Jorge Hernández and Samuel Castro González—ADS (Asociación
Demográfica Salvadoreña)
Jorge Odir Miranda—Asociación Atlacatl (AIDES)
Cristina Roque and Suzzane Calderón—Asociación de Mujeres
Flor de Piedra
Ricardo Arturo and Yolanda Barrientos—Fundación Olof Palme
Francisco Cartagena—Fundación Guadalupe
Julio Osegueda—FUNDASIDA

Guatemala

Annelise Salazar—Asociación de Salud Integral
Gustavo Castellanos Aragón—Centro de Desarrollo Humano de
Guatemala

Cristina Calderón—Fundación Preventiva del SIDA "Fernando Iturbe"
Hugo Valladares Morales—Asociación Gente Nueva
Erickson Chiclayo Salas-Cornejo—Asociación Gente Positiva
Rubén Mayorga Sagastume, María Antonieta Rodríguez, and Amarilis Barrios—OASIS

Honduras

Sadith Cáceres and Javier Cálix—PRODIM
Marco Antonio Alonza—Asociación Colectivo Violeta
Martha Manley Rodríguez—Gaviota
Rosa González—ASONAPVSIDAH

Mexico

Sandra Peniche Quintal—UNASSE
Javier Martínez Badillo—PTSC
Carlos García de León—AVE
Alicia Yolanda Reyes Alexánder—Amigos Previniendo el SIDA, A.C.
Juan Jacobo Hernández Chávez—Colectivo Sol, A.C., México

Nicaragua

Leonel Argüello Yrigoyen—CEPS
Norman Gutiérrez Morgan—Centro para la Prevención y Educación del SIDA
Rita Arauz—Fundación Nimehuatzin
Hazele Fonseca Navarro—Xochiquetzal
Flor de María Alvarado—ASONVIHSIDA
Ernesto López—Cruz Roja Nicaragüense
Edgar Jiménez Vargas
Pascual Orteills

Panama

Alfonso Lavergne and Elsi de Castillo—APLAFA
Maribel Coco and Lacina Méndez—ANADESAC
Orlando Quintero—Fundación Pro Bienestar y Dignidad de las
  Personas VIH/SIDA
Ricardo Beteta—Hombre y Mujeres de Panamá

Paraguay

Mirta Ruíz Díaz—Fundación VENCER
Ramón Martín Morán—REMAR Paraguay
Natalia Cerdido and Bernardo Puente—Grupo Luna Nueva
Manuel Fresco and Maura Villasanti—PREVER

Peru

Guido Mazzotti and Robinson Abello—Asociación Vía Libre
Domingo Cueto and Pablo Anamaría—PROSA
Aldo Araujo Neyra—Movimiento Homosexual de Lima
Carmen Murguia Pardo—Instituto de Educación y Salud
Julia Campos Guevara—Centro de Estudios con la Juventud
Eduardo Ticona Chávez—Hospital Nacional Dos de Mayo

Uruguay

Milka de Souza—FRANSIDA
María Luz Osimani and Juan José Meré —IDES
Patricia Ongay, Francisco Ottonelli, and María Salgado—
  IELSUR
Walter Florencio, Alvez Mariño, and Fernando Roccati—ATRU
Teresa Fernández Crepo and Magdalena Carrere—AMEPU
Rosario Viana and Susana Gerschuni Valmaggia—ASEPO

Venezuela

Feliciano Reyna—Acción Solidaria
Noris Ruiz—Agrupación de Mujeres Activistas Seropositivas
Norelia Albarrán and Bárbara Martínez—Fundación Marozo
Raiza Marín de Alizo—Resurrexit
Renate Koch and Edgar Carrasco—Acción Ciudadana Contra el
  SIDA (ACCSI)

Physicians

Argentina

Pedro Cahn—Fundación Huésped
Omar Sued—Hospital Fernández
Raúl Bortolozzi—Hospital Alberdi
Hugo Alberto Roland—Hospital Rawson
Víctor Bittar—Hospital Central, Mendoza

Bolivia

Ronald Andrade—Instituto Nacional de Laboratorios de Salud
Carlos Guachalla—Hospital Obrero
Saúl Pantoja—Caja Nacional de Salud

Brazil

Eduardo Sprinz—Hospital Petrópolis
Artur Kalicham—Hospital de São Paulo
David Uip—Hospital das Clínicas e INCOR
José Luiz de Andrade Neto—Curitiba
Cláudio Palombo—Centro Previdenciário de Niteroi
Rosana Del Bianco

Chile

Carlos Pérez Cortés—Fundación Arriarán
Erna Ripoll Moraga—Hospital Carlos Van Buren
Marcelo Wolf—Fundación Arriarán

Colombia

Guillermo Prada —Fundación Santafé
Berta Gómez—Clínica San Pedro Claver (Seguro Social)
Chantal Aristizábal—Hospital Central Policía Nacional
Otto Sussman—Hospital de San Ignacio

Costa Rica

Ricardo Boza Cordero—Hospital San Juan de Dios
María Paz León
Ignacio Salóm
Oscar Porras Madrigal—Clínica de Infección por VIH, Hospital
de Niños

Ecuador

Jacinto Vargas—Instituto Ecuatoriano de Seguridad Social
Richard Douce—Hospital Vozandes
Xavier Ochoa—Hospital Vicente Corral Moscoso
Fernando Mosquera—Hospital Carlos Andrade Marín

El Salvador

Jorge Panameño—Hospital de Especialidades del Seguro Social
José Ernesto Navarro Marín—Clínicas Médicas
Rolando Cedillos—Hospital Nacional Rosales
Joaquín Viana—Hospital de Ontología del Seguro Social
Mario Gamero—Hospital Benjamín Bloom

Guatemala

Carlos Rodolfo Mejía Villatoro—Hospital Roosevelt
Pedro Vilanueva Mirón—Infecto Centro
Eduardo Arathon—Hospital General San Juan de Dios

Honduras

Dennis Padgett Moncada—Instituto Hondureño de Seguro Social
F. Alvarado Matute
Norma Solórzano—Instituto Nacional de Tórax
Maribel Rivera Medina—Hospital Escuela

Mexico

Patricia Volkow
Samuel Ponce de León—Instituto Nacional de Ciencias Médicas y
  Nutrición
Carlos Ávila
Aurora Orzechowski Rallo
Noris Pavua Ruz—Clínica para Niños con Inmunodeficiencias,
  Universidad Nacional Autónoma de México

Nicaragua

Guillermo Porras
Carlos Quant

Panama

Xavier Saez Llorens—Hospital del Niño
Néstor Sosa—Royal Center

Paraguay

Perla Ortellado
Manuel Arbo
Adolfo Galeano—Instituto de Medicina Tropicala

Peru

Carlos Seas Ramos—Facultad de Medicina and Instituto de
  Medicina Tropical, Universidad Peruana Cayetano Heredia
José Ricardo Losno García—Clínica San Borja
Raúl Salazar Castro—Hospital Almenara
Pablo Grados Torres—Hospital María Auxiliadora
Luis Cuellar Ponce de León—Instituto Nacional de Neoplásica

Uruguay

Ignacio Mirazo—Servicio Enfermedades Infecto-Contagiosas
  "Dr. José Scosería"
Eduardo Savio—Facultad de Medicina—Universidad de la
  República
Pablo Cappucio—Hospital de Higiene

Venezuela

Regina López—Unidad de Immunosuprimidos, Dirección de
  Sanidad Fuerza Armada
Manuel Guzmán Blanco—Hospital Vargas de Caracas
María Eugenia Cavazza—Laboratorio CITOMED
Bernardo Vainrub—Hospital de Clínicas
Anselmo Rosales—Instituto Venezolano de los Seguros Sociales

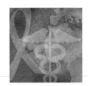

References

Adam, Barry D. 1993. "In Nicaragua: Homosexuality without a Gay World." *Journal of Homosexuality* 24:171–81.

Adams, K. Irene. 2000. "Ten Year Analysis of the Clinical AMMOR Street Kids Cohort: High Incidence of Risk Behaviour, Low Incidence of HIV Infection." *International Conference on AIDS* 13(1):404 (Abstract TuPeC3356).

Argentina, Ministerio de Salud, Unidad Coordinadora Ejecutiva VIH/SIDA y ETS. 2000. *Boletín sobre el SIDA en la República Argentina [Bulletin on AIDS in the Argentine Republic]*. Buenos Aires.

Ávila, M. M., E. Casanueva, C. Piccardo, and others. 1996. "HIV-1 and Hepatitis B Virus Infections in Adolescents Lodged in Security Institutes of Buenos Aires." *Pediatric AIDS and HIV Infection* 7:346–9.

Barbosa de Carvalho, Heráclito, Fabio Mesquita, Eduardo Massad, Regina Carvalho Bueno, Giselda Turienzo Lopes, Milton Arthur Ruiz, and Marcelo Nascimento Burattini. 1996. "HIV and Infections of Similar Transmission Patterns in a Drug Injector's Community of Santos, Brazil." *Journal of AIDS & Human Retroviruses* 12:84–92.

Barboza R., L. R. Pupo, A. Pluciennik, M. P. R. Oliveira, M. C. S. Monteiro, M. B. P. Melo, C. A. Santos, J. A. Lázaro, J. C. B. Pacca, and M. I. Nemes. 2000. "An Evaluation of Condom Distribution by Public Health System in the State of Sao Paulo, Brazil." *International Conference on AIDS* 13(2):514 (Abstract ThPeD5769).

Belo M., M. T. C. T. Belo, K. Sanches, A. Trajman, E. G. Teixeira, L. Selig, and M. M. Castello Branco. 2000. "Risk for Tuberculosis in AIDS Patients in Rio de Janeiro, Brazil." *International Conference on AIDS* 13(2):142 (Abstract WePeC4422).

Belza, María José, Alicia Llacer, Rocío Mora, María Morales, Jesús Castilla, and Luis De La Fuente. 2001. "Sociodemographic Characteristics and HIV Risk Behaviour Patterns of Male Sex Workers in Madrid, Spain." *AIDS Care* 13:677–82.

Bergenstrom, A., and L. Sherr. 2000. "A Review of HIV Testing Policies and Procedures for Pregnant Women in Public Maternity Units of Porto Alegre, Rio Grande do Sul, Brazil." *AIDS Care* 12:177–86.

Bolivia, Ministerio de Salud y Previsión Social, y PAHO. 2000a. *Diagnóstico de los Sistemas de Vigilancia Epidemiológica de VIH/SIDA/ITS del Área Andina [Diagnosis of HIV/AIDS Epidemiologic Surveillance Systems in the Andean Region].* La Paz.

Bolivia, Programa Nacional de ITS/SIDA. 2000b. *Plan Estratégico 2000–2004 de Prevención y Control de las Infecciones de Transmisión Sexual VIH-SIDA [Strategic Plan 2000–2004 for Prevention and Monitoring of HIV/AIDS Sexually Transmitted Infections].* La Paz.

Bueno, R., F. Mesquita, A. Kral, A. Reingold, M. Sanches, and I. Haddad. 2000. "Drug Using and Sexual Safety: Trends in the 1990s in Santos Metropolitan Region, Brazil." *International Conference on AIDS* 13(1):419 (Abstract TuPeC3429).

Burattini, M., E. Massad, M. Rozman, R. Azevedo, and H. Carvalho. 2000. "Correlation between HIV and HCV in Brazilian Prisoners: Evidence for Parenteral Transmission inside Prison." *Revista de Saúde Pública* 34:431–6.

Busza, Joanna R. 2001. "Promoting the Positive: Responses to Stigma and Discrimination in Southeast Asia." *AIDS Care* 13:441–56.

Cáceres, C. F., and P. Chequer. 2000. "Men Who Have Sex with Men and the HIV Epidemic in Latin America and the Caribbean." *International Conference on AIDS* 13(2):433 (Abstract ThOrD688).

Cáceres, Carlos F., Bárbara Vanoss Marín, and Esther Sid Hudes. 2000. "Sexual Coercion among Youth and Young Adults in Lima, Peru." *Journal of Adolescent Health* 27:361–7.

Cáceres, Carlos F., and Ana M. Rosasco. 1999. "The Margin Has Many Sides: Diversity among Gay and Homosexually Active Men in Lima." *Culture, Health & Sexuality* 1:261–75.

Cahn, P., W. H. Belloso, J. Murillo, and G. Prada-Trujillo. 2000. "AIDS in Latin America." *Infectious Disease Clinics of North America* 14(1):185–209.

Cano Flores, F. R., and L. F. Chávez Espina. 2000. "Implementation and Evaluation of an HIV/AIDS Prevention Program inside the Military Sector of Guatemala." *International Conference on AIDS* 13(2):500 (Abstract ThPeD5708).

Carpenter, Charles, Margaret A. Fischl, Scott M. Hammer, Martin S. Hirsch, Donna M. Jacobsen, David A. Katzenstein, Julio S. G. Montaner, Douglas D. Richman, Michael S. Saag, Robert T. Schooley, Melanie A. Thompson, Stefano Vella, Patrick G. Yeni, and Paul A. Volberding. 1998. "Antiretroviral Therapy for HIV Infection in 1998: Updated Recommendations of the International AIDS Society-USA Panel." *JAMA* 280:78–86.

Cartier, Luis, Fernando Araya, José Luis Castillo, Vladimir Zaninovic, Masanori Hayami, Tomoyuki Miura, Joko Imai, Shunro Sonoda, Hiroshi Shiraki, Kanji Miyamoto, and Kazuo Tajima. 1993. "Southernmost Carriers of HTLV-I/II in the World." *Japanese Journal of Cancer Research* 84:1–3.

Cartier, L., K. Tajima, F. Araya, and others. 1993. ["Preliminary Study of HTLV-I Seroprevalence in Chilean Indian Populations"]. *Revista Médica de Chile* 121:241–6.

Catania, Joseph, Dennis Osmond, Ronald D. Stall, Lance Pollack, Jay P. Paul, Sally Blower, Diane Binson, Jesse A. Canchola, Thomas C. Mills, Lawrence Fisher, Kyung-Hee Choi, Travis Porco, Charles Turner, Johnny Blair, Jeffrey Henne, Larry L. Bye, and Thomas C. Coates. 2001. "The Continuing HIV Epidemic among Men Who Have Sex with Men." *American Journal of Public Health* 91:907–14.

CDC (Centers for Disease Control and Prevention). 1987a. "Recommendations for Prevention of HIV Transmission in Health-Care Settings." *Morbidity and Mortality Weekly Report* 36(suppl. 2S):1S–18S.

———. 1987b. "Revision of the CDC Surveillance Case Definition for Acquired Immunodeficiency Syndrome." *Morbidity and Mortality Weekly Report* 26(suppl. 1):1–15.

———. 1988. "Update: Universal Precautions for Prevention of Transmission of Human Immunodeficiency Virus, Hepatitis B Virus, and Other Bloodborne Pathogens in Health-Care Settings." *Morbidity and Mortality Weekly Report* 37:377–88.

———. 1989. "Guidelines for Prevention of Transmission of Human Immunodeficiency Virus and Hepatitis B Virus to Health-Care and Public-Safety Workers." *Morbidity and Mortality Weekly Report* 38(S6):1–36.

———. 1992. "1993 Revised Classification System for HIV Infection and Expanded Surveillance Case Definition for AIDS among Adolescents and Adults." *Morbidity and Mortality Weekly Report* 41(RR-17):1–19.

———. 1999a. "Characteristics of Persons Living with AIDS at the End of 1997." *HIV/AIDS Surveillance Supplemental Report* 5(1):1–13.

———. 1999b. "Guidelines for National Human Immunodeficiency Virus Case Surveillance, Including Monitoring for Human Immunodeficiency Virus Infection and Acquired Immunodeficiency Syndrome." *Morbidity and Mortality Weekly Report* 48(RR13):1–27, 29–31.

———. 2001a. "Revised Guidelines for HIV Counselling, Testing and Referral" (Technical Expert Panel Review of CDC HIV counselling, testing and referral guidelines). *Morbidity and Mortality Weekly Report* 50(RR19):1–58.

———. 2001b. "Revised Recommendations for HIV Screening of Pregnant Women: Perinatal Counseling and Guidelines Consultation, April 26–27, 1999, Atlanta, Georgia." *Morbidity and Mortality Weekly Report* 50(RR19):59.

CDC, HIV/AIDS Prevention Research Synthesis Project. 1999. "Compendium of HIV Prevention Interventions with Evidence of Effectiveness." Atlanta, GA. Retrieved from www.cdc.gov/hiv/pubs/HIVcompendium.pdf.

Celantono, A., A. Ciliberti, S. Inchaurraga, A. Virgala, and C. Martearena. 2000. "Street Prostitution: Money vs. Use of Condoms." *International Conference on AIDS* 13:245 (Abstract WePeD4799).

Chile, Comisión Nacional del SIDA. 2000. *Boletín Epidemiológico Semestral VIH/SIDA [Weekly HIV/AIDS Epidemiologic Bulletin]* (No. 13). Ministerio de Salud, Santiago de Chile.

Cohen, Myron, and Joseph Eron. 2001. "Sexual HIV Transmission and Its Prevention." *Medscape HIV/AIDS Clinical Management Modules*. Retrieved March 7, 2001 from www.medscape.com.

Colombia, Ministerio de Salud, Dirección de Salud Pública; Instituto Nacional de Salud, Subdirección de Epidemiología y Laboratorio; and ONUSIDA. 2000. *Plan Estratégico de la Respuesta Nacional ante la Epidemia del VIH/SIDA, Años 2000–2003 [Strategic Plan for the National Response to the HIV/AIDS Epidemic, 2000–2003]*. Bogotá.

Costa Rica, Ministerio de Salud. 2001. *Plan Nacional Estratégico para el Abordaje Integral del VIH/SIDA 2001–2004 [National Strategic Plan for an Integrated Response to HIV/AIDS]*. San José.

Cymerman, P., A. Sánchez, G. Touze, D. Rossi, M. Vila, S. Ripski, and M. Nicolini. 2000. "Improving Injecting Drug Users' Access to Prevention through Pharmacies." *International Conference on AIDS* 13(2):251 (Abstract WePeD4825).

De Cock, Kevin W., and Anne M. Johnson. 1998. "From Exceptionalism to Normalisation: A Reappraisal of Attitudes and Practice around HIV Testing." *British Medical Journal* 316:290–3.

del Rio Zolezzi, Aurora, Ana Luisa Liguori, Carlos Magis-Rodríguez, José Luis Valdespino Gómez, María de Lourdes García García, and Jaime Sepúlveda Amor. 1995. "La Epidemia de VIH/SIDA y la Mujer en México" ["The HIV/ AIDS Epidemic and Women in México"]. *Salud Pública de México* 37:581–91.

Des Jarlais, Don C. 1995. "Harm Reduction—A Framework for Incorporating Science into Drug Policy." *American Journal of Public Health* 85(1):10–12.

Des Jarlais, Don C., Karl Dehne, and Jordi Casabona. 2001. "HIV Surveillance among Injecting Drug Users." *AIDS* 15(suppl. 3):S13–S22.

Des Jarlais, Don C., Holly H. Hagan, Samuel R. Friedman, Patricia Friedman, David Goldberg, Martin Frischer, Steven Green, Kerstin Tunving, Bengt Ljungberg, Alex Wodak, Michael Ross, David Purchase, Margaret E. Millson, and Ted Myers. 1995. "Maintaining Low HIV Seroprevalence in Populations of Injecting Drug Users." *JAMA* 274:1226–31.

Di Lonardo, M., N. C. Isola, M. Ambroggi, A. Rybko, and S. Poggi. 1995. "Mycobacteria in HIV-Infected Patients in Buenos Aires." *Tubercle and Lung Diseases* 76(3):185–89.

Díaz Lestrem, M., H. Fainboim, N. Méndez, and others. 1989. "HIV-1 Infection in Intravenous Drug Abusers with Clinical Manifestations of Hepatitis in the City of Buenos Aires." *Bulletin of the Pan American Health Organization* 23:35–41.

Díez, A. G., L. Grigaitis, A. M. Burgos, and N. Revsin. 2000. "[Buenos Aires] City Health Services: Obstacles in Early Detection, Treatment and Adherence." *International Conference on AIDS* 13(1):504 (Abstract TuPeD3722).

Drucker, Ernest, Peter Lurie, Alex Wodak, and Philip Alcabes. 1998. "Measuring Harm Reduction: The Effects of Needle and Syringe Exchange Programs and Methadone Maintenance on Ecology of HIV." *AIDS* (suppl. A):S217–30.

Duenas-Barajas, Eduardo, Jaime Eduardo Bernal, Dihanna R. Vaught, Vivek R. Nerurkar, Piedad Sarmiento, Richard Yanagihara, and D. Carleton Gajdusek. 1993. "Human Retroviruses in Amerindians of Colombia: High Prevalence of Human T Cell Lymphotropic Virus Type II Infection among the Tunebo Indians." *American Journal of Tropical Medicine and Hygiene* 49:657–63.

Dunn, John, and Ronaldo R. Laranjeira. 1999. "Transitions in the Route of Cocaine Administration—Characteristics, Direction and Associated Variables." *Addiction* 94:813–24.

Echevarría, J. M., L. Blitz-Dorfman, and F. H. Pujot. 1996. ["Infection by Hepatitis Virus among the Indigenous Populations of South America: A Review of the Problem"]. *Investigación Clínica* 37:191–200.

Ecuador, Ministerio de Salud Pública, and WHO. 2000. *Diagnóstico de los Sistemas de Vigilancia Epidemiológica de VIH/SIDA/ITS del Área Andina, Ecuador*. Quito.

Egger, Matthias, Josefina Pauw, Athanasios Lopatatzidis, Danilo Medrano, Fred Paccaud, and George Davey Smith. 2000. "Promotion of Condom Use in a High-Risk Setting in Nicaragua: A Randomized Controlled Trial." *Lancet* 355:2101–5.

El Salvador, Ministerio de Salud Pública y Asistencia Social. 2001. *Plan Nacional de Prevención y Control de ITS/VIH/SIDA 2001–2003 [National Plan for the Prevention and Monitoring of STIs/HIV/AIDS]* (draft). San Salvador.

European Centre for the Epidemiological Monitoring of AIDS. 1993. "1993 Revision of the European AIDS Surveillance Case Definition." *HIV/AIDS Surveillance in Europe Quarterly Report* no. 37:23–28.

———. 1995. "European Case Definition for AIDS Surveillance in Children Revision 1995." *HIV/AIDS Surveillance in Europe Quarterly Report* no. 48:46–53.

Ferri, Cleusa P., and Michael Gossop. 1999. "Route of Cocaine Administration: Patterns of Use and Problems among a Brazilian Sample." *Addictive Behaviors* 24:815–21.

Fleming, Douglas T., and Judith N. Wasserheit. 1999. "From Epidemiological Synergy to Public Health Policy and Practice: The Contribution of Other Sexually Transmitted Diseases to Sexual Transmission of HIV Infection." *Sexually Transmitted Infections* 75:3–17.

Frasca, T., B. C. Flores, C. Serrano, P. Berendsen, and G. Guajardo. 2000. "Needs Assessment for HIV Prevention among Gay-Bisexual Men in Three Provincial Capitals of Chile." *International Conference on AIDS* 13(2):436 (Abstract ThOrD736).

Fundación Mexicana de la Salud, SIDALAC (Iniciativa Regional sobre SIDA para América Latina y el Caribe), ONUSIDA, and Comisión Europea. 2002. *Indicadores Financieros de las Respuestas Nacionales contra el VIH/SIDA: Estimaciones 2002 [Financial Indicators of the National Responses to HIV/AIDS: 2002 Estimates]*. Mexico, D.F.

García, R., W. Klaskala, Y. Pena, and M. K. Baum. 2000. "Behavioral Change Intervention for Women at Low and High Risk for STD/HIV in Colombia." *International Conference on AIDS* 13(2):405 (Abstract ThPeC5347).

García-García, M. L., M. E. Jiménez-Corona, A. Ponce de León, A. Jimenez-Corona, M. Palacios-Martínez, S. Balandrano-Campos, L. Ferreyra-Reyes, L. Juarez-Sandino, J. Sifuentes-Osornio, H. Olivera-Díaz, J. L. Valdespino-Gomez, and P. M. Small. 2000. "Mycobacterium Tuberculosis Drug Resistance in a Suburban Community in Southern Mexico." *International Journal of Tuberculosis and Lung Disease* 4:S168–70.

German, Robert R. 2000. "Sensitivity and Predictive Value Positive Measurements for Public Health Surveillance Systems." *Epidemiology* 11:720–7.

Ghys, Peter, Mamadou Diallo, Virginie Ettiegne-Traoré, Glen A. Satten, Camille K. Anoma, Chantal Maurice, Jean Claude Kadjo, Issa-Malik Coulibaly, Stefan Z. Wiktor, Alan E. Greenberg, and Merie Laga. 2001. "Effect of Interventions to Control Sexually Transmitted Disease on the Incidence of HIV Infection in Female Sex Workers." *AIDS* 15:1421–31.

Ghys, Peter D., Carol Jenkins, and Elisabeth Pisani. 2001. "HIV Surveillance among Female Sex Workers." *AIDS* 15(suppl. 3):S33–S40.

Grande, M. A. 2000. "Risk Perceptions and Practices of Sexual Street Workers about STDs, HIV/AIDS in Lima, Peru." *International Conference on AIDS* 13(2):249 (Abstract WePeD4814).

Guatemala, Grupo Temático Ampliado de ONUSIDA. 2000. *Plan Integrado en Apoyo al Plan Estratégico Nacional de VIH/SIDA.* Guatemala City.

Guatemala, Ministerio de Salud Pública y Asistencia Social. 1999. *Plan Estratégico Nacional ITS/VIH/SIDA 1999–2003.* Guatemala City.

Halperin, Daniel. 1998. "HIV, STDs, Anal Sex and AIDS Prevention Policy in a Northeastern Brazilian City." *International Journal of STDs and AIDS* 9:294–8.

Halperin, Daniel. 1999. "Heterosexual Anal Intercourse: Prevalence, Cultural Factors and HIV Infection and Other Health Risks, Part I." *AIDS Patient Care and STDs* 13:717–30.

Hammer, Scott M., Kathleen E. Squires, Michael D. Hughes, Janet Grimes, Lisa M. Demeter, Judith S. Currier, Joseph J. Eron, Judith E. Feinberg, Henry H. Balfour, Lawrence R. Deyton, Jeffrey A. Chodakewitz, Margaret A. Fischl, John P. Phair, Louise Pedneault, Bach-Yen Nguyen, and Jon C. Cook, for the AIDS Clinical Trials Group 320 Study Team. 1997. "A Controlled Trial of Two Nucleoside Analogues Plus Indinavir in Persons with Human Immunodeficiency Virus Infection and CD4 Cell Counts of 200 per Cubic Millimeter or Less." *New England Journal of Medicine* 337:725–33.

Hartgers, Christina, Ernst C. Buning, Gerrit Van Santen, Annette D. Verster, and Roel A. Coutinho. 1989. "Impact of the Needle and Syringe Exchange Program in Amsterdam in Injecting Risk Behavior." *AIDS* 3:571–6.

HIV and AIDS in the Americas: An Epidemic with Many Faces. 2001. Geneva, Switzerland: UNAIDS, WHO, and PAHO. Retrieved from www.census.gov/ipc/www/hivaidinamerica.pdf.

Honduras, Ministerio de Salud Pública. 1999. *Plan Estratégico Nacional de Lucha contra el SIDA 1998–2001 [National Strategic Plan to Fight against HIV/AIDS].* Tegucigalpa.

Hudgins, Rebekah, Jane McCusker, and Anne Stoddard. 1995. "Cocaine Use and Risky Injection and Sexual Behaviors." *Drug and Alcohol Dependence* 37:7–14.

Hughes, Gwenda, with Kholoud Porter and O. Nöel Gill. 1998. "Indirect Methods for Estimating Prevalence of HIV Infections: Adults in England and Wales at the End of 1993." *Epidemiology and Infection* 121:165–72.

Hughes, Patrick. 1977. *Behind the Wall of Respect: Community Experiments in Heroin Addiction Control.* Chicago: University of Chicago Press.

Inciardi, James A. 1996. "HIV Risk Reduction and Service Delivery Strategies in Criminal Justice Settings." *Journal of Substance Abuse Treatment* 13:421–8.

Inciardi, James A., and Hilary L. Surratt. 1998. "Children in the Streets of Brazil: Drug Use, Crime, Violence and HIV Risks." *Substance Use and Misuse* 33: 1461–8.

International Perinatal HIV Group. 1999. "The Mode of Delivery and the Risk of Vertical Transmission of Human Immunodeficiency Virus Type 1." *New England Journal of Medicine* 340:977–87.

Izazola-Licea, J. Antonio, Carlos Ávila Figueroa, Carlos Cáceres Palacios, Bilali Camara, André Nunes, Jorge A. Saavedra López, Manuel Sierra, and Abel Víquez, eds. 1998. *Situación Epidemiológica y Económica del SIDA en América Latina y el Caribe.* Mexico, D.F.: Fundación Mexicana de la Salud.

Jha, Prabhat, Lara M. E. Vaz, Francis Plummer, Nico J. D. Nagelkerke, Bridget Willbond, Elizabeth N. Ngugi, Stephen Moses, Grace John, Ruth Nduatr, Kelly McDonald, and Seth Berkley. 2001. "The Evidence Base for Interventions to Prevent HIV Infection in Low and Middle Income Countries" (CMH Working Paper Series, Paper No WG5:2). Available at http://www3.who.int/whosis/cmh/cmh_papers/e/pdf/wg5_paper02.pdf.

Jorge, S., K. Russell, C. Carcamo, M. Negrete, A. Paredes, R. Galván, and M. Chiappe. 2000. "HIV Sentinel Surveillance for Men Who Have Sex with Men in Peru." *International Conference on AIDS* 13(2):381 (Abstract ThOrC717).

Kalichman, A. O., M. C. Gianna, R. A. Souza, S. M. H. S. Bueno, N. J. S. Santos, A. A. Maldonado, F. N. Dias, and J. B. A. Souza. 2000. "Evaluating the Impact of Availability of ARV Therapy in an STD/AIDS Referral and Training Center, Sao Paulo, Brazil." *International Conference on AIDS* 13(2):418 (Abstract ThPeC5408).

Kaplan, Edward H., Kaveh Khoshnood, and Robert Heimer. 1994. "A Decline in HIV Infected Needles Returned to the New Haven Needle Exchange Program: Client Shift or Needle Exchange?" *American Journal of Public Health* 84: 1991–4.

Karon, John M., with Meena Khare and Philip S. Rosenberg. 1998. "The Current Status of Methods for Estimating the Prevalence of Human Immunodeficiency Virus in the United States of America." *Statistical Medicine* 17:127–42.

Kegeles, Susan, Robert Hays, Lance Pollack, and Thomas Coates. 1999. "Mobilizing Young Gay and Bisexual Men for HIV Prevention: A Two-Community Study. *AIDS* 13:1753–62.

Kelly, Jeffrey. 2000. "HIV Prevention Interventions with Gay or Bisexual Men and Youth." *AIDS* 14(suppl. 2):S34–S39.

Kerr-Pontes, Ligia, Rogelio Gondim, Rosa S. Mota, Telma A. Martins, and David Wypij. 1999. "Self-Reported Sexual Behaviour and HIV Risk Taking among Men Who Have Sex with Men in Fortaleza, Brazil." *AIDS* 13:709–17.

Klein, Charles. 1999. "'The Ghetto Is Over, Darling': Emerging Gay Communities and Gender and Sexual Politics in Contemporary Brazil." *Culture, Health & Sexuality* 1:239–59.

Krieger, James, Chesa Collier, Lin Song, and Donald Martin. 1999. "Linking Community-Based Blood Pressure Measurement to Clinical Care: A Randomized Controlled Trial of Outreach and Tracking by Community Health Workers." *American Journal of Public Health* 89:856–61.

Kupek, Emil J. 2001. "The Reduction of HIV Transfusion Risk in Southern Brazil in the 1990s." *Transfusion Medicine* 11(2):75–8.

Laufer, Franklin N. 2001. "Cost-Effectiveness of Syringe Exchange as an HIV Prevention Strategy." *Journal of Acquired Immune Deficiency Syndrome* 28:273–8.

León, Pilar, Evaristo Venegas, Loreto Bengoechea, Ernesto Rojas, José López, Consuelo Elola, and José M. Echevarría. 1999. "Prevalencia de las Infecciones por Virus de la Hepatitis B, C, D y E en Bolivia" ["Prevalence of Infections by Hepatitis B, C, D and E Viruses in Bolivia"]. *Revista Panamericana de Salud Pública* 5:144–51.

Levine, William, Rita Revollo, Verónica Kaune, Juan Vega, Freddy Tinajeros, Marcela Garnica, Miguel Estensoro, Joel Lewis, Guimar Higueras, Raquel Zurita, Linda Wright-De Agüero, Reynaldo Pareja, Patricia Miranda, Raymond L. Ransom, Akbar A. Zaidi, María Luisa Melgar, and Joel N. Kuritsky. 1998. "Decline in Sexually Transmitted Disease Prevalence in Female Bolivian Sex Workers: Impact of an HIV Prevention Project." *AIDS* 12:1899–1906.

Libonatti, O., E. Lima, A. Peruga, R. González, F. Zacarías, and M. Weissenbacher. 1993. "Role of Drug Injection in the Spread of HIV in Argentina and Brazil." *International Journal of STDs and AIDS* 4:135–41.

Lima, Elson S., Samuel R. Friedman, Francisco I. Bastos, Paulo R. Telles, Patricia Friedman, Thomas P. Ward, and Don des Jarlais. 1994. "Risk Factors for HIV-1 Seroprevalence among Drug Injectors in the Cocaine-Using Environment of Rio de Janeiro. *Addiction* 89:689–98.

London, Andrew S., and Arodys Robles. 2000. "The Co-occurrence of Correct and Incorrect HIV Transmission Knowledge and Perceived Risk for HIV among Women of Childbearing Age in El Salvador." *Social Sciences and Medicine* 51:1267–78.

Loo Méndez, E., G. Hernández Tepichini, and X. Terán Toledo. 2000. "STI/HIV/AIDS in Male and Female Sex Workers in a Center of Integral Attention in Mexico." *International Conference on AIDS* 13(2):428 (Abstract ThPeC5456).

Low, Nicola, Matthias Egger, Anna Gorter, Peter Sandiford, Alcides González, Johanna Pauw, Jane Ferrie, and George Davey Smith. 1993. "AIDS in Nicaragua: Epidemiological, Political, and Sociocultural Perspectives." *International Journal of Health Services* 23:685–702.

Ludo, S., H. Ligorio, E. Careno, S. Guerrero, D. Lavarello, M. Agostini, and J. Palazzi. 2000. "HIV Detection [Campaign] in Rosario City, Argentina." *International Conference on AIDS* 13(2):420 (Abstract ThPeC5416).

MacNeil, Joan M., and Sandra Anderson. 1998. "Beyond the Dichotomy: Linking HIV Prevention with Care." *AIDS* 12(suppl. 2):S19–S26.

Magis-Rodríguez, Carlos, Aurora del Rio Zolezzi, José Luis Valdespino Gómez, and María de Lourdes García. 1995. "Casos de SIDA en el Área Rural de México" ["AIDS Cases in Rural Areas of Mexico"]. *Salud Pública de México* 37:615–23.

Maidagan C., L. Echegoy, A. Tesolini, F. Garat, M. Hernández, E. Lucero, L. Trape, M. A. Acosta, and M. Agostini. 2000. "HIV Prevention and Testing Project for the Inmates at the Police Stations of Rosario, Argentina." *International Conference on AIDS* 13(1):495 (Abstract TuPeD3677).

Manock, Stephen R., Patricia M. Kelley, Kenneth C. Hyams, Richard Douce, Roger D. Smalligan, Douglas M. Watts, Trueman W. Sharp, John L. Casey, John L. Gerin, Ronald Engle, Aracely Alava-Alprecht, Carlos Mosquera Martínez, Narcisa Brito Bravo, Angel Gustavo Guevara, Kevin L. Russel, Wilson Mendoza, and Carlos Vimos. 2000. "An Outbreak of Fulminant Hepatitis Delta in the Waorani, an Indigenous People of the Amazon Basin of Ecuador." *American Journal of Tropical Medicine and Hygiene* 63:209–13.

Massad, E., M. Rozman, R. S. Azevedo, A. S. B. Silveira, K. Takey, Y. I. Yamamoto, L. Strazza, M. M. C. Ferreira, H. B. Carvalho, and M. N. Burattini. 1999. "Seroprevalence of HIV, HCV and Syphilis in Brazilian Prisoners: Preponderance of Parenteral Transmission." *European Journal of Epidemiology* 15:439–45.

McCarthy, Michael C., F. Stephen Wignall, Jorge Sánchez, Eduardo Gotuzzo, Jorge Alarcón, Irving Phillips, Douglas M. Watts, and Kenneth Hyams. 1996. "The Epidemiology of HIV-1 Infection in Peru, 1986–1990." *AIDS* 10:1141–5.

McFarland, Willi, and Carlos Cáceres. 2001. "HIV Surveillance among Men Who Have Sex with Men." *AIDS* 15(suppl. 3):S23–S32.

Medeot, Silvia, Silvia Nates, Alejandra Recalde, Sandra Gallego, Eduardo Maturano, Miguel Giordano, Horacio Serra, Juan Reategui, and Cesar Cabezas. 1999. "Prevalence of Antibody to Human T Cell Lymphotropic Virus Types 1/2 among Aboriginal Groups Inhabiting Northern Argentina and the Amazon Region of Peru." *American Journal of Tropical Medicine and Hygiene* 60:623–9.

Merson, Michael H., Julia Dayton, and Kevin O'Reilly. 2000. "Effectiveness of HIV Prevention Interventions in Developing Countries." *AIDS* 14(suppl. 2): S69–S84.

Mesquita, Fabio, Alex Kral, Arthur Reingold, Regina Bueno, Daniela Trigueiros, and Paula J. Araujo. 2001. "Trends of HIV Infection among Injection Drug Users in Brazil in the 1990s: The Impact of Changes in Patterns of Drug Use." *Journal of Acquired Immune Deficiency Syndrome* 28:298–302.

Mexico, Secretaría de Salud, CONASIDA. 2002. "Las Cifras del SIDA en México" ["AIDS Statistics in México"]. Retrieved from http://www.ssa.gob.mx/conasida/.

Michaud, Catherine M., Cristopher J. Murray, and Barry R. Bloom. 2001. "Burden of Disease—Implications for Future Research. *JAMA* 285:535–9.

Miguez-Burbano, M. J., I. Angarita, J. M. Shultz, G. Shor-Posner, W. Klaskala, J. L. Duque, H. Lai, B. Londono, and M. K. Baum. 2000. "HIV-Related High Risk Sexual Behaviors among Women in Bogota, Colombia." *Women & Health* 30(4):109–19.

Miranda, A., M. Alves, R. Neto, E. Andriolo, and K. R. Areal. 2000. "Seroprevalence and Risk Factors for HIV, HBV and Syphilis in Women at Their First Visit to the Antenatal Clinics." *International Conference on AIDS* 13(2):135 (Abstract WePeC4392).

Miranda, Angélica E., Paulo M. Vargas, Michael E. St. Louis, and María Carmen Viana. 2000. "Sexually Transmitted Diseases among Female Prisoners in Brazil: Prevalence and Risk Factors." *Sexually Transmitted Diseases* 27:491–5.

Murray, Cristopher J. L., and Alan D. Lopez. 1998. *Health Dimensions of Sex and Reproduction*. Geneva, Switzerland: World Health Organization.

Nasiff, V., M. Beltran, R. Gil, A. Reniero, and N. Sanga. 2000. "TBC and HIV Infection: A 12 Year Experience at San Isidro Municipal Hospital, Buenos Aires, Argentina." *International Conference on AIDS* 13(2):138 (Abstract WePeC4404).

National Institute on Drug Abuse. 2000. *The NIDA Community-Based Outreach Model: Manual to Reduce the Risk of HIV and Other Blood-Borne Infections in Drug Users* (NIH publication no. 00-4812). Bethesda, MD.

National Institutes of Health, Consensus Development Conference Statement. 2000. "February 11–13, 1997: Interventions to Prevent HIV Risk Behaviors." *AIDS* 14(suppl. 2):S85–S95.

Nelles, J., A. Fuhrer, H. P. Hirsbrunner, and T. W. Harding. 1998. "Provision of Syringes: The Cutting Edge of Harm Reduction in Prison?" *British Medical Journal* 317:270–3.

Nicaragua, Ministerio de Salud. 2000. *Plan Estratégico Nacional de Lucha contra ETS/VIH/SIDA, Nicaragua, 2000–2004 [National Strategic Plan to Fight STIs/HIV/SIDA]*. Managua.

Onorato, Ida M., with T. Stephen Jones and Willis R. Forrester. 1990. "Using Seroprevalence Data in Managing Public Health Programs." *Public Health Report* 105:163–6.

ONUSIDA (Programa Conjunto de las Naciones Unidas sobre el VIH/SIDA). 1997a. "Las Cárceles y el SIDA: Punto de vista del ONUSIDA, abril de 1997" ["Prisons and AIDS: UNAIDS Position, April 1997"] (Best Practice Collection). Geneva, Switzerland. Retrieved from www.unaids.org.

———. 1997b. "Educación sobre el SIDA en la Escuela" ["AIDS Education in Schools"] (Technical Update, Best Practice Collection). Geneva, Switzerland. Retrieved from www.unaids.org.

———. 1998. "Guía para la Planificación Estratégica de una Respuesta Nacional al VIH/SIDA" ["Guide to Strategic Planning for a National Response to HIV/AIDS"]. Geneva, Switzerland. Retrieved from www.unaids.org.

———. 2000a. "Análisis de la Situación de la Epidemia del VIH/SIDA y de la Respuesta Nacional en Bolivia" ["Analysis of the State of the HIV/AIDS Epidemic and the National Response in Bolivia"]. La Paz, Bolivia.

———. 2000b. "El Género y el VIH/SIDA" ["Gender and HIV/AIDS"] (Technical Update, Best Practice Collection). Geneva, Switzerland. Retrieved from www.unaids.org.

Organista, Kurt C., Pamela Organista, J. E. García de Alba, and others. 1997. "Survey of Condom-Related Beliefs, Behaviors, and Perceived Social Norms in Mexican Migrant Laborers." *Journal of Community Health* 22(3):185–98.

Organización Mundial de Salud and ONUSIDA. 2000. "Guías sobre la Vigilancia del VIH de Segunda Generación" ["Guidelines for Second-Generation AIDS Surveillance"] (WHO/CDS/CSR/EDC/2000.5). Geneva, Switzerland.

Ortiz-Mondragen, R. I., L. Pedrosa-Islas, M. Mendoza, V. Rozenel, and C. Magis. 2000. "Do Young People Have Access to Condoms in Mexico City?" *International Conference on AIDS* 13(1):490 (Abstract TuPeD3654).

Osmond, Dennis, with Andrew B. Bindman, Karen Vranizan, Stan Lehman, Frederick M. Hecht, Dennis Keane, and Arthur Reingold, for the Multistate Evaluation of Surveillance for HIV Study Group. 1999. "Name Based Surveillance and Public Health Interventions for Persons with HIV Infection." *Annals of Internal Medicine* 131:775–9.

PAHO (Pan American Health Organization). 1990. "Working Group on AIDS Case Definition." *Epidemiological Bulletin* 10(4):9–11.

———. 1999. "Fortalecimiento de los Bancos de Sangre en la Región de las Américas" ["Strengthening of Blood Banks in the Latin American Region"] (Documento de trabajo CD41/19). San Juan, Puerto Rico.

———. 2000a. *Building Blocks: Proceedings of the Consultation on Standards of Care for Persons Living with HIV/AIDS in the Americas.* Washington, D.C.

———. 2000b. *Final Report: Retreat on Blood Safety.* Antigua, Guatemala. Retrieved from http://www.paho.org/English/HSP/HSE/HSE06/bloodsafety-lab01-2000.pdf.

————. 2000c. *Vigilancia del SIDA en las Américas—Informe Bianual de Mayo 2000 [AIDS Surveillance in the Americas—Biannual Report of May 2000]*. Retrieved from www.paho.org/Spanish/HCP/HCA/report_may_2000.pdf.

————. 2001a. *AIDS Surveillance in the Americas: Biannual Report (Draft)*. Retrieved from www.paho.org/english/HCP/HCA/final_bulletin_dec01.pdf.

————. 2001b. "Estimates of Incidence and Prevalence of STIs among Adults in Latin America and the Caribbean." Unpublished presentation. Washington, D.C.

Palella, Frank J., Kathleen M. Delaney, Anne C. Moorman, Mark O. Loveless, Jack Fuhrer, Glen A. Satten, Diane J. Aschman, and Scott D. Holmberg, for the HIV Outpatient Study Investigators. 1998. "Declining Morbidity and Mortality among Patients with Advanced Human Immunodeficiency Virus Infection." *New England Journal of Medicine* 338:853–60.

Panama, Ministerio de Salud. 1999. *Plan Nacional de Salud Sexual y Reproductiva [National Plan for Sexual and Reproductive Health]*. Panama City.

Pando, M. de los A., S. Gianni, H. Salomon, M. Negrete, K. L. Russell, L. Martínez Peralta, J. K. Karr, and M. M. Ávila. 2000. "Risk Behavior of HIV-1 Infected Maternity Patients and Their Sexual Partners in Buenos Aires, Argentina." *International Conference on AIDS* 13(1):429 (Abstract TuPeC3471).

Pappaioanou, Marguerite, with Timothy J. Dondero, Lyle R. Petersen, Ida M. Onorato, Carolyn D. Sanchez, and James W. Curran. 1990. "The Family of HIV Seroprevalence Surveys: Objectives, Methods and Uses of Sentinel Surveillance for HIV in the United States." *Public Health Report* 105:163–6.

Park, I., D. Morisky, C. Sneed, and S. Alvear. 2000. "Correlates of HIV Risk among Ecuadorian Adolescents." *International Conference on AIDS* 13(2):216 (Abstract WePeD4667).

Pauw, Johanna, Jane Ferrie, Rosaura Rivera Villegas, Josefina Medrano Martínez, Anna Gorter, and Matthias Egger. 1996. "A Controlled HIV/AIDS-Related Health Education Programme in Managua, Nicaragua." *AIDS* 10:537–44.

Pedrola, M., J. Giagnorio, G. Cortez, N. Azcona, A. Sponer, and M. Giagnorio. 2000. "Risk Factors for the Infection of HIV in Adolescents Who Take Illegal Drugs and Are at Secondary School in Four Public Schools from Venado Tuerto." *International Conference on AIDS* 13(2):115 (Abstract WePeC4302).

Peru, Grupo Temático de la Naciones Unidas. 2001. *Primer Plan Estratégico Integrado del Grupo Temático de las Naciones Unidas sobre VIH/SIDA/Peru [First Integrated Strategic Plan of the United Nations Working Group on HIV/AIDS in Peru]*. Lima.

Piot, Peter, and Awa M. Coll. 2001. "International Response to the HIV/AIDS Epidemic: Planning for Success." *Bulletin of the World Health Organization* 79:1106–12.

Rich, Josiah D., Leah Holmes, Cristopher Salas, Grace Macalino, Deborah Davis, James Ryczek, and Timothy Flanigan. 2001. "Successful Linkage of Medical Care and Community Services for HIV Positive Offenders Being Released from Prison." *Journal of Urban Health* 78:279–89.

Rodríguez, M. A., R. Mayorga, S. Álvarez, A. García, K. Foreit, C. Núñez, and E. Zelaya. 2000. "A Qualitative Study of Sexual Behaviors, Social Norms, Human Rights and Risk Contexts for HIV Infection in Men Who Have Sex with Men (MSM) in Downtown Guatemala City." *International Conference on AIDS* 13(2):235 (Abstract WePeD4752).

Rotheram-Borus, Mary Jane, Susan Cantwell, and Peter A. Newman. 2000. "HIV Prevention Programs with Heterosexuals." *AIDS* 14(suppl. 2):S59–S67.

Ruiz, Mónica S., Alicia R. Gable, Edward H. Kaplan, Michael A. Stoto, Harvey V. Fineberg, and James Trussel, eds. 2000. *No Time To Lose: Getting More from HIV Prevention.* Washington, D.C.: National Academy Press. Retrieved from www.nap.edu.

Sabin, Keith M., Robert L. Frey, Rosemary Horsley, and Stacie M. Greby. 2001. "Characteristics and Trends of Newly Identified HIV Infections among Incarcerated Populations: CDC HIV Voluntary Counseling, Testing, and Referral System, 1992–1998." *Journal of Urban Health* 78:241–55.

Samayoa, B., M. Martínez, T. Velásquez, Z. Fuentes Urrutia, and J. M. Ramírez. 2000. "Using a Rapid Test in Counseling HIV Testing Services in Guatemalan Urban Clinic." *International Conference on AIDS* 13(1):380 (Abstract TuOrC306).

Sanches, K., A. Trajman, and E. G. Teixeira. 2000. "Increasing Frequency of Elderly among AIDS Patients in Rio de Janeiro, Brazil." *International Conference on AIDS* 13(1):396 (Abstract TuPeC3321).

Sánchez, J., J. Ojeda, P. García, A. Paredes, C. Carcamo, J. Bernales, R. Galván, J. Campos, K. Russell, C. Celum, M. Negrete, and K. Holmes. 2000. "Incidence and Risk Factors for HIV Acquisition among Men Who Have Sex with Other Men: The Alaska Cohort of Lima." *International Conference on AIDS* 13(1):409 (Abstract TuPeC3380).

Sánchez Pérez, Héctor Javier, and D. Halperin Frisch. 1997. "Retos a Superar en el Control de la Tuberculosis Pulmonar en la Región Fronteriza de Chiapas, México" ["Obstacles to Overcome in the Control of Pulmonary Tuberculosis in the Border Region of Chiapas, Mexico"]. *Gaceta Sanitaria* 11:281–6.

Scalway, Thomas. 2001. "Young Men and HIV: Culture, Poverty and Sexual Risk" (Panos Report No. 41). Geneva, Switzerland, and London, England: UNAIDS and The Panos Institute. Retrieved from www.panos.org.uk.

Schmunis, Gabriel A., Fabio Zicker, Francisco Pinheiro, and David Brandling-Bennett. 1998. "Risk for Transfusion-Transmitted Infectious Diseases in Central and South America." *Emerging Infectious Diseases* 4(1):5–11.

Schwartlander, Bernhard, Peter D. Ghys, Elisabeth Pisani, Sonja Kiessling, Stefano Lazzari, Michael Carael, and John M. Kaldor. 2001. "HIV Surveillance in Hard-to-Reach Populations." *AIDS* 15(suppl. 3):S1–S3.

Sepúlveda Amor, Jaime, Aurora del Rio Zolezzi, José Luis Valdespino Gómez, María de Lourdes García García, Liliana Velásquez Velásquez, and Patricia Volkow. 1995. "La Estrategia de Prevención de Transmisión del VIH/SIDA a través de la Sangre y Sus Derivados en México" ["Strategy to Prevent HIV/AIDS Transmission through Blood and Blood Products in Mexico"]. *Salud Pública de México* 37:624–35.

Serra, M., J. Russi, J. Viñoles, M. T. Pérez, M. Negrete, K. L. Russell, J. K. Carr, and M. Weissenbacher. 2000. "Prevalence of HIV-1, Risk Behavior and Genetic Epidemiology of Transvestite Commercial Sex Workers in Montevideo, Uruguay." *International Conference on AIDS* 13(1):389 (Abstract TuPpC1176).

Sonoda, Shunro, Hong Chuai Li, Luis Cartier, Lautaro Nunez, and Kazuo Tajima. 2000. "Ancient HTLV Type 1 Provirus DNA of Andean Mummy." *AIDS Research and Human Retroviruses* 16:1753–6.

Soto, R., I. Epinoza, R. Meza, N. Aldana, A. Sevilla, A. Guillén, S. Jiménez, M. Baum, and N. Amador. 2000. "Epidemiological Profile, HIV Incidence, and Retention Rates in a Cohort of Female Sex Workers in Honduras: Preliminary Results." *International Conference on AIDS* 13(2):380 (Abstract ThOrC676).

Stimson, Gerry V., Gail Eaton, Tim Rhodes, and Robert Power. 1994. "Potential Development of Community Oriented HIV Outreach among Drug Injectors in the UK." *Addiction* 89:1601–11.

Summers, Todd, Freya Spielberg, Chris Collins, and Thomas Coates. 2000. "Voluntary Counselling, Testing and Referral for HIV: New Technologies, Research Findings Create Dynamic Opportunities." *Journal of Acquired Immune Deficiency Syndrome* 25(suppl. 2):S128–35.

Surratt, Hilary L. 2000. "Indigence, Marginalization and HIV Infection among Brazilian Cocaine Users." *Drug and Alcohol Dependence* 58:267–74.

Surratt, H., J. Inciardi, F. Pechansky, and L. von Diemen. 2000. "Regional Differences in HIV Risk among Cocaine Injectors in Two Brazilian Cities." *International Conference on AIDS* 13(1):392 (Abstract TuPpC1250).

Thacker, S. B., with S. Redmond, R. B. Rothemberg, S. B. Spitz, K. Choi, and M. C. White. 1986. "A Controlled Trial of Disease Surveillance Strategies." *American Journal of Preventive Medicine* 2:345–50.

Trotter, Robert T., Anne M. Bowen, and James Potter, Jr. 1995. "Network Models for HIV Outreach and Prevention Programs for Drug Users." In R. Needle, S. Genser, and R. Trotter, eds., *Social Networks, Drug Abuse and HIV Transmission* (NIDA Research Monograph no. 151). Rockville, MD.: U.S. Department of Health and Human Services.

UNAIDS (Joint United Nations Programme on HIV/AIDS). 1997a. "Impact of HIV and Sexual Health Education on the Sexual Behaviour of Young People: A Review Update" (Best Practice Collection). Geneva, Switzerland. Retrieved from www.unaids.org.

———. 1997b. "Learning and Teaching about AIDS at School" (Technical Update). Geneva, Switzerland. Retrieved from www.unaids.org.

———. 1999a. "Counselling and Voluntary Testing for Pregnant Women in High HIV Prevalence Countries: Elements and Issues" (Best Practice Collection). Geneva, Switzerland. Retrieved from www.unaids.org.

———. 1999b. "Prevention of HIV Transmission from Mother to Child: Strategic Options" (Best Practice Collection). Geneva, Switzerland. Retrieved from www.unaids.org.

———. 2000a. "AIDS and Men Who Have Sex with Men" (Best Practice Collection). Geneva, Switzerland. Retrieved from www.unaids.org.

———. 2000b. "Argentina: Epidemiological Fact Sheet on HIV/AIDS and Sexually Transmitted Infections, 2000 Update." Geneva, Switzerland. Retrieved from http://www.unaids.org/hivaidsinfo/statistics/fact_sheets/index_en.htm.

———. 2000c. "Bolivia: Epidemiological Fact Sheet on HIV/AIDS and Sexually Transmitted Infections, 2000 Update." Geneva, Switzerland. Retrieved from http://www.unaids.org/hivaidsinfo/statistics/fact_sheets/index_en.htm.

———. 2000d. "Brazil: Epidemiological Fact Sheet on HIV/AIDS and Sexually Transmitted Infections, 2000 Update." Geneva, Switzerland. Retrieved from http://www.unaids.org/hivaidsinfo/statistics/fact_sheets/index_en.htm.

————. 2000e. "Chile: Epidemiological Fact Sheet on HIV/AIDS and Sexually Transmitted Infections, 2000 Update." Geneva, Switzerland. Retrieved from http://www.unaids.org/hivaidsinfo/statistics/fact_sheets/index_en.htm.

————. 2000f. "Colombia: Epidemiological Fact Sheet on HIV/AIDS and Sexually Transmitted Infections, 2000 Update." Geneva, Switzerland. Retrieved from http://www.unaids.org/hivaidsinfo/statistics/fact_sheets/index_en.htm.

————. 2000g. "Consultation on STD Interventions for Preventing HIV: What Is the Evidence?" (Best Practice Collection). Geneva, Switzerland. Retrieved from www.unaids.org.

————. 2000h. "Costa Rica: Epidemiological Fact Sheet on HIV/AIDS and Sexually Transmitted Infections, 2000 Update." Geneva, Switzerland. Retrieved from http://www.unaids.org/hivaidsinfo/statistics/fact_sheets/index_en.htm.

————. 2000i. "Ecuador: Epidemiological Fact Sheet on HIV/AIDS and Sexually Transmitted Infections, 2000 Update." Geneva, Switzerland. Retrieved from http://www.unaids.org/hivaidsinfo/statistics/fact_sheets/index_en.htm.

————. 2000j. "El Salvador: Epidemiological Fact Sheet on HIV/AIDS and Sexually Transmitted Infections, 2000 Update." Geneva, Switzerland. Retrieved from http://www.unaids.org/hivaidsinfo/statistics/fact_sheets/index_en.htm.

————. 2000k. "Epidemiological Fact Sheets on HIV and Sexually Transmitted Infections, 2000 (updated)." Geneva, Switzerland. Retrieved from http://www.unaids.org/hivaidsinfo/statistics/factsheets/index.

————. 2000l. "Female Sex Worker HIV Prevention Projects: Lessons Learnt from Papua New Guinea, India and Bangladesh" (Case Study). Geneva, Switzerland.

————. 2000m. "Guatemala: Epidemiological Fact Sheet on HIV/AIDS and Sexually Transmitted Infections, 2000 Update." Geneva, Switzerland. Retrieved from http://www.unaids.org/hivaidsinfo/statistics/fact_sheets/index_en.htm.

————. 2000n. *Guidelines for Second Generation HIV Surveillance.* Geneva, Switzerland.

————. 2000o. "Honduras: Epidemiological Fact Sheet on HIV/AIDS and Sexually Transmitted Infections, 2000 Update." Geneva, Switzerland. Retrieved from http://www.unaids.org/hivaidsinfo/statistics/fact_sheets/index_en.htm.

————. 2000p. "Mexico: Epidemiological Fact Sheet on HIV/AIDS and Sexually Transmitted Infections, 2000 Update." Geneva, Switzerland. Retrieved from http://www.unaids.org/hivaidsinfo/statistics/fact_sheets/index_en.htm.

————. 2000q. "Nicaragua: Epidemiological Fact Sheet on HIV/AIDS and Sexually Transmitted Infections, 2000 Update." Geneva, Switzerland. Retrieved from http://www.unaids.org/hivaidsinfo/statistics/fact_sheets/index_en.htm.

————. 2000r. "Panama: Epidemiological Fact Sheet on HIV/AIDS and Sexually Transmitted Infections, 2000 Update." Geneva, Switzerland. Retrieved from http://www.unaids.org/hivaidsinfo/statistics/fact_sheets/index_en.htm.

————. 2000s. "Paraguay: Epidemiological Fact Sheet on HIV/AIDS and Sexually Transmitted Infections, 2000 Update." Geneva, Switzerland. Retrieved from http://www.unaids.org/hivaidsinfo/statistics/fact_sheets/index_en.htm.

————. 2000t. "Peru: Epidemiological Fact Sheet on HIV/AIDS and Sexually Transmitted Infections, 2000 Update." Geneva, Switzerland. Retrieved from http://www.unaids.org/hivaidsinfo/statistics/fact_sheets/index_en.htm.

————. 2000u. "Preventing the Transmission of HIV among Drug Abusers: A Position Paper of the United Nations System." Geneva, Switzerland. Retrieved from www.unaids.org.

————. 2000v. "Putting Knowledge to Work: Technical Resource Networks for Effective Response to HIV/AIDS" (Best Practice Collection). Geneva, Switzerland. Retrieved from www.unaids.org.

————. 2000w. *Report on the Global HIV/AIDS Epidemic.* Geneva, Switzerland.

————. 2000x. "The Role of Name-Based Notification in Public Health and HIV Surveillance" (Best Practices Collection). Geneva, Switzerland. Retrieved from www.unaids.org.

————. 2000y. "Uruguay: Epidemiological Fact Sheet on HIV/AIDS and Sexually Transmitted Infections, 2000 Update." Geneva, Switzerland. Retrieved from http://www.unaids.org/hivaidsinfo/statistics/fact_sheets/index_en.htm.

————. 2000z. "Venezuela: Epidemiological Fact Sheet on HIV/AIDS and Sexually Transmitted Infections, 2000 Update." Geneva, Switzerland. Retrieved from http://www.unaids.org/hivaidsinfo/statistics/fact_sheets/index_en.htm.

————. 2001a. "Drug Abuse and HIV/AIDS: Lessons Learned" (Case Studies booklet). Geneva, Switzerland. Retrieved from www.unaids.org.

————. 2001b. *The Global Strategy Framework on HIV/AIDS.* Geneva, Switzerland.

————. 2001c. "The Impact of Voluntary Counseling and Testing: A Global Review of the Benefits and Challenges" (Best Practice Collection). Geneva, Switzerland. Retrieved from www.unaids.org.

UNAIDS, the Prince of Wales Business Leaders Forum, and the Global Business Council on HIV and AIDS. 2000. *The Business Response to HIV/AIDS: Impact and Lessons Learned.* Geneva, Switzerland. Retrieved from www.unaids.org.

United Nations. 2000. "Preventing the Transmission of HIV among Drug Abusers: A Position Paper of the United Nations System." Retrieved from www.unaids.org.

Uribe Zúñiga, Patricia, Griselda Hernández-Tepichin, Carlos del Rio Chiriboga, and Víctor Ortiz. 1995. "Prostitución y SIDA en la Ciudad de México" ["Prostitution and AIDS in Mexico City"]. *Salud Pública de México* 37:592–601.

van Ameijden, Erik J. C., John K. Watters, J. Anneke van den Hoek, and Roel A. Coutinho. 1995. "Interventions among Injecting Drug Users: Do They Work?" *AIDS* 9(suppl. A):S75–S84.

Venezuela, República Bolivariana de, Ministerio de Salud y Desarrollo Social. 2001. *Plan Estratégico Nacional ITS/VIH/SIDA 2002–2004* (draft). Caracas.

Viana, M., S. Gerschuni, and C. Dos Santos. 2000. "Violations of Human Rights of PLWH within Uruguayan Prisons." *International Conference on AIDS* 13(1):433 (Abstract TuOrD321).

Vicente, Ana C., Koko Otsuki, Nelson B. Silva, Marcia C. Castilho, Flavio S. Barros, Danuta Pieniazek, Dale Hu, Mark A. Rayfield, Gustavo Bretas, and Amilcar Tanuri. 2000. "The HIV Epidemic in the Amazon Basin Is Driven by Prototypic and Recombinant HIV-1 Subtypes B and F." *Journal of Acquired Immune Deficiency Syndrome* 23:327–31.

Volkow, Patricia, José Rogelio Pérez-Padilla, Carlos del Rio, and Alejandro Mohar. 1998. "The Role of Commercial Plasmapheresis Banks on the AIDS Epidemic in Mexico." *Revista de Investigación Clínica* 50(3):221–6.

Weinhardt, Lance S., Michael P. Carey, Blair T. Johnson, and Nicole L. Bickham. 1999. "Effects of HIV Counseling and Testing on Sexual Risk Behavior: A Meta-Analytic Review of Published Research 1985–1997." *American Journal of Public Health* 89:1397–1405.

Wheeler, David A., Eduardo G. Arathoon, Michael Pitts, Rolando A. Cedillos, T. Efrain Bu, Guillermo D. Porras, Gisela Herrera, and Nestor R. Sosa. 2001. "Availability of HIV Care in Central America." *JAMA* 286:853–60.

Wood, Evan, Marck W. Tyndall, Patricia M. Spittal, Katty Li, Thomas Kerr, Robert S. Hogg, Julio S. G. Montaner, Michael V. O'Shaughnessy, and Martin T. Schechter. 2001. "Unsafe Injection Practices in a Cohort of Injection Drug

Users in Vancouver: Could Safer Injecting Rooms Help?" *Canadian Medical Association Journal* 165:405–10.

World Bank. 1997. *Confronting AIDS: Public Priorities in a Global Epidemic.* Oxford, England: Oxford University Press.

———. 2001. "Thailand's Response to AIDS: Building on Success, Confronting the Future." Washington, D.C. Retrieved from www.worldbank.org.

World Health Organization. 1986. "Provisional WHO Clinical Case Definition for AIDS." *Weekly Epidemiological Record* 61(10):72–3.

Zacarías, F., R. S. González, P. Cuchi, A. Yanez, A. Peruga, R. Mazin, C. Betts, and M. Weissenbacher. 1994. "HIV/AIDS and Its Interaction with Tuberculosis in Latin America and the Caribbean." *Pan American Health Organization Bulletin* 28:312–23.

Zapiola, I., S. Salomone, A. Alvarez, M. C. Scolastico, R. A. Koessel, J. Lemus, C. Wainstein, and G. Muchinik. 1996. "HIV-1, HIV-2, HTLV-I/II and STD among Female Prostitutes in Buenos Aires, Argentina." *European Journal of Epidemiology* 12(1):27–31.

Zuloaga Posada, Luz, Cecilia Soto Vélez, and Diva Jaramillo Vélez. 1995. "Comportamiento Sexual y Problemas de Salud en Adultos Jóvenes, Universidad de Antioquia, 1991" ["Sexual Behavior and Health Problems in University Students, University of Antioquia, 1991"]. *Pan American Health Organization Bulletin* 29:299–311.

Zurita, Susana, Cecilia Costa, Douglas Watts, Sonia Indacochea, Pablo Campos, Jorge Sánchez, and Eduardo Gotuzzo. 1997. "Prevalence of Human Retroviral Infection in Quillabamba and Cuzco, Peru: A New Endemic Area for Human T Cell Lymphotropic Virus Type 1." *American Journal of Tropical Medicine and Hygiene* 56:561–5.

Zwarenstein, Merrik. 2001. "Commentary: Sputum Prevalence Data Suggest Mexican TB Rates Will Explode on Contact with HIV Epidemic." *International Journal of Epidemiology* 30:393.

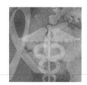

Index

Note: f indicates figures and t indicates tables

199–201; Paraguay, 247–49; Peru, 230–31; Uruguay, 253–55; Venezuela, 212–13
prisoners and HIV, 68; intervention campaigns, 98–99, 100t, 147; prevention efforts (*see* prevention issues and challenges by country)

República Bolivariana de Venezuela. *See* Venezuela

sexually transmitted infections (STIs): contribution to epidemic, 8, 9t; interventions needed, 144–45; prevalence rates, 65, 68
social and legal restrictions on homosexuality, 109–10, 111t
Southern Cone: Argentina, 39–41; Chile, 42–43; Paraguay, 41; primary mode of transmission, 36, 37f; Uruguay, 42. *See also specific countries*
STIs. *See* sexually transmitted infections
surveillance: active vs. passive, 54–56; allocation of resources and personnel, 51–52; of behavior, 69–71; blood safety and, 74–75, 76f; case definition, 52–54, 55t; case identification, 57–59; case reporting, 54, 56f; challenges for, 79–80, 154–55; country status (*see* surveillance issues and challenges by country); data distribution to health professionals, 62–64; forms of case identification, 49; HIV diagnosis services availability, 71–72; HIV testing and diagnosis costs, 73; HIV testing frequency, 74; importance of, 50–51; intervention campaigns needed, 156; legislation regarding confidentiality issues, 59; need for improvement, 76–77; notification delays, 60–62; population analysis, 65, 68–69; prevalence rates in low-risk groups, 69, 70t; quality and validity of available information, 49–50, 65; reporting forms, 56–57; sentinel surveillance utility, 64–65, 66–67t; strengths of current programs, 77–78; systems evaluation, 64; underreporting, 60–62
surveillance issues and challenges by country: Argentina, 244–45; Bolivia, 238–39;

Brazil, 208–9; Chile, 262–63; Colombia, 220–21; Costa Rica, 196–97; Ecuador, 226–27; El Salvador, 178–79; Guatemala, 172–73; Honduras, 184–86; Mexico, 166–67; Nicaragua, 190–91; Panama, 202–3; Paraguay, 250–51; Peru, 232–33; Uruguay, 256–57; Venezuela, 214–15

testing programs for HIV: access to, 116–18, 119f; cost and availability problems, 148, 150; diagnosis costs and, 73; frequency of use, 74; laboratory infrastructure problems, 149–50
tuberculosis (TB) co-morbidity with HIV, 2–3, 8

UNAIDS (Joint United Nations Programme on HIV/AIDS), 1, 4
Uruguay: blood safety issues and challenges, 257; care issues and challenges, 255; epidemic status, 252–53; epidemiology of epidemic, 42; funding resources, 253; key problems, 253; prevention issues and challenges, 253–55; surveillance issues and challenges, 256–57

Venezuela, República Bolivariana de: blood safety issues and challenges, 215; care issues and challenges, 213–14; epidemic status, 210; epidemiology of epidemic, 28, 30–31; funding resources, 211; key problems, 211; prevention issues and challenges, 212–13; surveillance issues and challenges, 214–15
vertical transmission. *See* women and HIV

women and HIV: feminization of epidemic, 5, 15–16; gender distribution of AIDS cases, 15–16; intervention campaigns, 147–48; mother-to-child transmission prevention, 113–14, 115f, 150; prevention efforts (*see* prevention issues and challenges by country)
World Health Organization (WHO), 1, 4

youths. *See* adolescents and youths